AAK-8217

OXFORD MEDICAL PUBLICATIONS

Unexplained Infertility

Unexplained Infertility

Patrick J. Taylor

Professor of Obstetrics and Gynaecology,
University of British Columbia, and
Chairman of Obstetrics and Gynaecology,
St Paul's Hospital, Vancouver, Canada

John A. Collins

Professor and Chairman,
Department of Obstetrics and Gynaecology,
McMaster University, Ontario, Canada

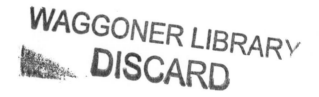
OXFORD   NEW YORK   TOKYO
OXFORD UNIVERSITY PRESS
1992

Oxford University Press, Walton Street, Oxford OX2 6DP
Oxford   New York   Toronto
Delhi   Bombay   Calcutta   Madras   Karachi
Petaling Jaya   Singapore   Hong Kong   Tokyo
Nairobi   Dar es Salaam   Cape Town
Melbourne   Auckland
and associated companies in
Berlin   Ibadan

Oxford is a trade mark of Oxford University Press

Published in the United States
by Oxford University Press, New York

A catalogue record for this book is available from the British Library

Library of Congress Cataloging in Publication Data
Taylor, Patrick J.
Unexplained infertility / Patrick J. Taylor, John A. Collins.
p.   cm.
1. Infertility.   2. Infertility—Psychological aspects.
I. Collins, John A., 1933–   .
RC889.T33   1992   616.6'92—dc20   92–23032
ISBN 0–19–262290–0

Typeset by
Footnote Graphics, Warminster, Wilts
Printed and bound in Great Britain
by Biddles Ltd, Guildford and King's Lynn

Blessed trinity have pity,
You can give the blind man sight,
Fill the barren rocks with grasses,
Grant this house a child tonight.

(11th century, author unknown;
translated from the original Irish)

Contents

Acknowledgement

Much of the material used in this book has been derived from information collected during the Canadian Infertility Therapy Evaluation Study (CITES). We wish to thank most sincerely our co-investigators in the study. Their names and centres are listed here. William Wrixon, MD, Halifax, Nova Scotia; Rodolphe Maheux, MD, and Nacia Faure, MD, Laval, Québec; Togas Tulandi, MD, and D. Robert A. McInnes, MD, Montréal, Québec; John F. Jarrel, MD, Hamilton, Ontario; R. Hugh Gorwill, MD, and Robert L. Reid, MD, Kingston, Ontario; David C. Cumming, MD, and Josef Z. Scott, MB, Edmonton, Alberta; Timothy C. Rowe, MB, and Peter F. McComb, MB, Vancouver, British Columbia; H. Anthony Pattinson, MB, and Arthur Leader, MD, Calgary, Alberta; John McCoshen, Ph.D., and Ronald A. Livingston, MB, Winnipeg, Manitoba; John E. H. Spence, MD, and Peter Garner, MB, Ottawa, Ontario; Charles W. Simpson, MD and David R. Poplin, MD, Saskatoon, Saskatchewan; Serge Belisle, MD, and Youssef AinMelk, MD, Sherbrooke, Québec; Stanley E. Brown, MD, and Earl R. Plunkett, MD, London, Ontario, Canada.

Supported by the National Research and Development Program, Project Number 6606-2628-44, National Department of Health and Welfare, Ottawa, Canada.

1 Introduction

'A reputation for curing sterility is spoken of as if it were founded on substantial claims. As in other departments of therapeutics, there has been a great failure of logic. The *post-hoc* and *propter-hoc* have been confused, a coincidence has been regarded as a consequence, and the credulity of patients and doctors alike has been the basis for useless and injurious practice.' This statement was made by J. Matthews Duncan in 1883. Despite the impressive advances made in our understanding of reproductive physiology and the introduction of new diagnostic and therapeutic approaches for the infertile couple, much of this failure of logic persists today. Nowhere is this more apparent than in the enigma of unexplained infertility. Consensus on the definition of unexplained infertility and its rational treatment is, understandably but sadly, lacking.

The diagnosis of unexplained infertility is one of exclusion, and depends upon the accurate use of investigations of the reproductive processes. To be effective, such clinical investigations must have a sound basis in the physiology of reproduction. The physician must constantly question the value of any proposed test, inquiring as to its validity and accuracy, and ultimately, as to whether or not it will alter the outcome of any proposed management.

Management of unexplained infertility will depend in each case upon the individual needs of the couple. Infertility is the inability to conceive a wanted child. While this statement is accurate, it does not truly address the complexity of the childless state. Why do some patients consult a physician after six months, others wait five years, and still others seek no medical advice at all? Why does minimal intervention satisfy some couples, while others insist on treatment after treatment after treatment? The answer must be one of individual need.

A more complete description of infertility must encompass not only childlessness and the obvious desire to conceive, but also the needs of the couple for:

- autonomy;
- accurate answers to their questions;
- emotional support; and
- if conception does not occur, the feeling that all reasonable avenues have been explored.

When no cause for the infertility has been detected, it is more difficult to provide the couple with answers, to give back to them some control of their destiny, and to offer them the best chance of successful conception. Any proposed treatment must be empirical, as the nature of the causative defect is not understood. When treatment is to be offered, the proposed approach should offer a higher likelihood of pregnancy than would no formal medical intervention. An understanding of the prognosis for untreated couples and of the efficacy of empirical treatment allows such decisions to be made.

For those unfortunate enough not to conceive, the inevitable uncertainty about the cause inhibits their ability to feel they have given it their 'best shot'. Emotional healing is very personal. Couples need their physician to be available, to offer support and sympathy when it is most required, to provide information, and to dispel the myths surrounding human reproduction.

THE PRESENT BOOK: TOPICS COVERED AND ORDER OF TREATMENT

This monograph will formulate a preliminary definition of unexplained infertility, and consider the prevalence of the condition. A more accurate working clinical definition will be developed one step at a time from a critical appraisal of the physiology of reproduction and of certain pathological states and their investigation.

Conception and the successful establishment of pregnancy require the following series of events:

(1) ovulation and endometrial preparation for implantation;
(2) spermatogenesis and sperm transport in the male;
(3) sperm transport and oocyte transport in the female; and
(4) fertilization and early embryonic development.

The physiology and investigation of each will be described.

Whether endometriosis, immunological phenomena, infection, or uterine lesions can inhibit conception is very unclear. Current ideas on each of these subjects will be discussed, and the methods of investigating these potential causes of infertility will be scrutinized. At the conclusion of each chapter in this section of the monograph a definition of unexplained infertility in its relation to the potentially adverse condition considered in that chapter will be formulated.

These chapters will lead to a short chapter summarizing the relevant information into a working definition of unexplained infertility and the investigations necessary to establish the diagnosis. Once this definition is established, the management of the condition will be considered, with particular attention to the prognosis for untreated couples, the likely emotional impact on the couple, the efficacy of empirical treatment, and a guide to clinical decision-making.

When it is recognized that infertility will affect 1.2 couples per 1000 of the population annually (Hull *et al*. 1985), and that 1 in every 6 couples will at some time consult a specialist with concerns about their perceived infertility, it rapidly becomes apparent that involuntary childlessness is a problem of significant magnitude. It is hoped that what follows will be of help to the physician in providing the best possible service in meeting the diagnostic needs of infertile couples in general, and the therapeutic needs of those in whom a diagnosis of unexplained infertility has been made.

2 Overview of the prevalence of unexplained infertility and the investigations necessary to make the diagnosis

Before 1900 virtually all cases of infertility were unexplained. From 1900 to 1940 major advances occurred in the diagnosis of tubal, seminal, and ovulatory disorders. Non-surgical evaluation of tubal patency first became available in 1920, when Rubin described the oxygen insufflation test; and, within a year, carbon dioxide replaced oxygen as the gas of choice (Rubin 1921).

The first evaluation of the ejaculate was reported by Macomber and Sanders (1929). They correlated the occurrence of pregnancy in couples who were infertile with systematic counting of living spermatozoa in the male partners' ejaculates. Azoospermia and oligozoospermia were found to contribute to infertility. The authors suggested that the lower level of normal sperm density should be 60 million per millilitre—a criterion which has subsequently been revised.

A diagnosis of ovulatory dysfunction was dependent upon a clinical history of amenorrhoea until Rubenstein (1937) correlated changes in vaginal smears with a thermal shift in the basal body temperature. Rock and Bartlett (1937) used histological examination of endometrial tissue both as presumptive evidence that ovulation was occurring and as a method of timing ovulation. By 1937, a couple would have been defined as suffering from unexplained infertility if, after a reasonable passage of time, no abnormalities were detected through the measurement of basal temperature, endometrial biopsy, semen analysis, or tubal insufflation. In the 1990s many more sophisticated tests, of more or less value, have been

Table 2.1 *English-language reports on the proportion of infertility clinic patients with unexplained infertility*

Decade of report	Number of couples	Proportion with Unexplained Infertility (95 per cent CI)*	Authors
1950s	134	13 (7,19)	Frank 1950
	658	5 (3,7)	Johansson 1957
	1437	31 (29,33)	Southam and Buxton 1957
Subtotal	2229	22	
1960–79	500	13 (10,16)	Raymont *et al.* 1969
	644	22 (19,25)	Newton *et al.* 1974
	512	18 (15,21)	Dor *et al.* 1977
Subtotal	1656	18	
1980s	1020	0 (13,23)	Harrison 1980
	196	18 (4,10)	Sorensen 1980
	291	7 (20,28)	Thomas and Forrest 1980
	583	1 (0,2)	Insler *et al.* 1981
	400	24 (20,28)	West *et al.* 1982
	141	11 (6,16)	Verkauf 1983
	493	26 (22,30)	Kliger 1984
	708	24 (21,27)	Hull *et al.* 1985
	1297	13 (11,15)	Collins *et al.* 1986
Subtotal	5129	14	
Total	9014	17	

* CI: confidence interval

added. Yet a dilemma remains, because in many couples none of these investigations reveal a cause.

In order to arrive at a preliminary definition, it would seem germane to examine the prevalence of unexplained infertility as described in clinical studies. Not surprisingly, the reported prevalence is very variable, ranging from 0 to 31 per cent of couples investigated. Table 2.1 demonstrates the observed prevalence in several studies from the last forty years, and Fig. 2.1 illustrates how other diagnoses are distributed. Although there is an apparent reduction in the extent of the condition in the later reports, this trend disappears if the two studies with the lowest and highest percentages are excluded. Variability in the reported percentages

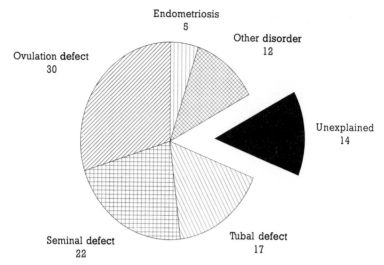

Fig. 2.1 *Prevalence of unexplained infertility and other infertility diagnoses (numbers are per cent of couples). Reports 1980 and later, 5129 couples. References: Table 2.1.*

arises from the nature of the patient population studied and from the extent of the investigation performed before a final diagnosis was made. Referral patterns vary widely. Even in a single multi-centre study, the proportion of unexplained infertility ranged from 8 to 38 per cent (Collins and Rowe 1989).

The extent of which diagnostic investigations will be performed may be affected by the wishes of the couple, their availability to attend for the performance of certain tests, and the protocol followed by the particular unit or practitioner. The last will be dependent upon the clinician's perception of the published experience and personal preferences. The availability of certain procedures will vary from unit to unit, and may be heavily biased in favour of a particular clinical or research interest. These factors lead to differences among centres in the minimum investigations required to diagnose unexplained infertility (Table 2.2). In these reports only the semen analysis was an absolute prerequisite; but a reasonable minimal requirement for the investigation of the infertile couple before the diagnosis of unexplained infertility is made would also include

Table 2.2 *Diagnostic protocols in 20 studies reporting pregnancy rates among couples with unexplained infertility*

Diagnostic test	Test required (No. of studies)*
Semen analysis	20
Endometrial biopsy or serum progesterone estimation	19
Laparoscopy	16
Hysterosalpingogram	13
Postcoital test	13
Sperm-directed antibody tests	1

* Details and references in Table 12.1

confirmation of ovulation and evaluation of the femal genital tract, including tubal patency.

The infertile couple and their medical advisers are constantly under pressure to 'do something'; and the first 'something' to be done is to arrange a series of investigations. The true value of any such investigation is whether or not it can predict with reasonable accuracy the fertility potential of an individual couple. For example, it is highly unlikely that conception will occur if the male partner is found to be azoospermic. The situation is much less clear if the results of semen analysis are normal or somewhat abnormal. If it is felt that such a patient should be evaluated further, none of the current battery of tests of sperm function define *in vivo* fertilizing ability. It is possible, in part, to assess the ability of spermatozoa to penetrate cervical mucus, undergo capacitation and the acrosome reaction, and penetrate the zona pellucida. Other aspects of sperm function critical to the successful initiation of pregnancy are not amenable to study. And while some of these procedures may improve our understanding of the physiology of the spermatozoon, subsequent chapters will examine how well (or poorly) these investigations predict future fertility. Similar difficulties bedevil the assessment of the absolute occurrence and quality of ovulation. Moreover, while the patency of the fallopian tubes can be tested, little insight can be gained into the function of these organs *in vivo*.

The diagnosis of unexplained infertility is one of exclusion. If a true cause of infertility can be identified, then by definition un-explained infertility cannot exist. How well the newer investigations serve this purpose and help to refine the definition will be explored in more detail in the following eight chapters.

A more accurate preliminary definition of unexplained infertility can be formulated in general terms as follows: 'unexplained infertility can be said to exist when all tests of the reproductive processes which are reliable in identifying those conditions that can be shown to impair fertility are normal'.

The definition will require constant reappraisal as new testing procedures are validated. But until every facet of the reproductive process is completely understood and amenable to accurate investi-gation the dilemma will remain: does unexplained infertility repre-sent a '. . . misfortune due to the laws of chance or a limitation of our knowledge' (Southam 1960)?

3 The physiology and investigation of ovulation and endometrial preparation for implantation

INTRODUCTION

A prerequisite for successful pregnancy is the release of a mature oocyte. This chapter will consider the physiology of ovulation and related events, and how they are best investigated. From this information, that aspect of the definition of unexplained infertility that pertains to the ovulatory process will be derived.

THE PHYSIOLOGY OF FEMALE GAMETOGENESIS

The development and release of a mature oocyte are dependent upon an elaborately orchestrated synchrony between the ovary and the higher endocrine centres. Although the hypothalamus and pituitary are important, it is now clear that the chief regulatory organ is the Graafian follicle. The hormones and other factors produced by the ovary are responsible for the cyclic changes which occur in the endometrium from one menstrual period to the next. The biosynthesis, metabolism, and laboratory measurement of the reproductive hormones are beyond the scope of this text. Those wishing to pursue the fundamental endocrinology in depth are referred to Edwards (1980), Speroff *et al.* (1989*a*), and Yen and Jaffe (1986).

This section will:

- describe the anatomical events occurring within the ovary;
- describe the events occurring within the hypothalamus and pituitary; and

- show how follicular and hypothalamic pituitary events interact to cause reproductive steroid hormone production and ovulation.

The primordial follicle

The ovaries are paired organs, lying behind the broad ligaments, suspended laterally by the ovarian ligament and medially by the suspensory ligament. They are devoid of peritoneal covering. Each has a cortex and a medulla, and it is within the stroma of the cortex that the oocytes and their surrounding cells, the granulosa and theca, lie.

Primitive germ cells migrate to the embryonic ovary by the fifth week of embryonic life (Baker 1981). Between six and eight weeks there is rapid mitotic multiplication of the oogonia. Meiotic division begins at 15 weeks, and the oogonia become primary oocytes (Manotaya and Potter 1963). The first meiotic division is arrested in prophase, and the oocytes remain in a state of suspended animation until further maturation occurs. At 20 weeks, the presence of the oocyte stimulates the organization of a single layer of mesenchymal and epithelial cells—the granulosa—which surrounds the oocyte. This layer of cells and the oocyte constitute the primordial follicle (Speroff *et al.* 1989*b*).

The primordial follicles begin a process of maturation. The process starts *in utero*, and ceases when the supply of primordial follicles is exhausted—a phenomenon which occurs at the time of the menopause. Eighty per cent of all primordial follicles are lost during fetal life, and many more by the process of atresia from birth until the onset of ovulatory cycles.

Follicular maturation

Once reproductive maturity has been achieved (usually 8 to 24 months after menarche) follicular maturation may lead to ovulation or atresia, processes that occur in cyclic fashion throughout the reproductive life of a woman. The intraovarian events in such cycles are the focus of this section. These events concern the development of a group, or cohort, of primordial follicles.

Initial growth of the primordial follicles occurs independently of any hormonal stimulus, and will progress to atresia unless the appropriate hormonal stimulus occurs. This is termed recruitment of a cohort of follicles (Vermesh and Kletsky 1987). As the hormonal milieu changes, one follicle from the cohort will gain dominance in the early days of the cycle, go on to ovulate, and form the corpus luteum. The rest will achieve varying degrees of maturation before succumbing to atresia. At the beginning of a menstrual cycle, a cohort of follicles is recruited. The dominant follicle will progress successfully through three stages:

- pre-antral,
- antral, and
- pre-ovulatory.

Ovulation will occur, and this follicle will become the corpus luteum.

The *pre-antral follicle* can be recognized by the enlargement of its oocyte and the appearance of the zona pellucida, a species-specific membrane which surrounds the oocyte. The granulosa cells become multilayered, and the surrounding stroma becomes organized into the theca. The pre-antral follicles synthesize and release oestrogens, which are formed by the aromatization of androgenic precursors. Both growth and aromatization, and hence oestrogen production, are dependent on follicle stimulating hormone (FSH), which is released from the pituitary.

The local effects of the oestrogen and FSH induce production of fluid. This fluid accumulates in a cavity—the antrum. The *antral follicle* is surrounded by theca. The granulosa lying within the theca surround the antrum, at the pole of which is the oocyte, also surrounded by granulosa. Those cells immediately adjacent to the oocyte begin to form the cumulus mass, the innermost layers of which form the corona radiata.

The follicular fluid provides a hormonal environment particular to each oocyte. Whereas an oestrogenic milieu is beneficial, an androgenic milieu in the follicular fluid will produce degenerative changes in the oocytes (Erickson *et al.* 1985). Levels of oestrogen in the follicular fluid reflect FSH activity. At this period, the production of oestrogen is rising. In addition, the presence of oestrogen in the follicle increases the number of FSH receptors in the granulosa. The most oestrogenic follicle and, hence, the one with the best ability to use the available FSH, outstrips the rest of the cohort and gains dominance on about the fifth day of the cycle (Chikazawa *et al.* 1986). As the dominant follicle develops, the vasculature to its theca increases, and, by the ninth day, has become twice that of the other follicles.

The ovulatory process is triggered by a surge of luteinizing hormone (LH). To respond, the follicle must possess receptors for LH. FSH induces the development of these LH receptors in the larger antral follicles. This action is obligatorily mediated by oestrogen.

In addition to the interaction of the peptide and steroid hormones, local growth factors, which include transforming growth factor, epidermal growth factor, fibroblast growth factor, angiogenic growth factor, platelet-derived growth factor, and insulin-like growth factor, are also important at unspecified stages of follicular development (Speroff *et al.* 1989*b*). The follicular fluid contains proteins—in particular inhibin, which also controls follicular growth by modifying FSH production (De Jong and Sharpe 1976).

As ovulation approaches, the antral follicle continues to grow, and becomes recognizable as the *pre-ovulatory follicle*. The theca is very vascular, and the cells contain vacuoles. Lipid inclusions appear in the enlarged granulosa cells. This process of luteinization begins as early as the tenth day, at which time production of progesterone begins. Thus progesterone synthesis begins before ovulation, and is not only a post-ovulatory event (Aedo *et al.* 1976).

The physical appearances of the follicle have by now changed. That portion lying within the ovarian cortex is vascularized, surrounded by smooth muscle fibres and several thick layers of theca and luteinized granulosa. The portion lying above the surface of the ovary is thin, in places consisting of a single layer of granulosa cells. The oocyte, which has completed the first meiotic division and formed the first polar body, lies within the cumulus mass attached to the wall of the follicle. The diameter of the pre-ovulatory follicle, measured ultrasonographically, is about 2.2 cm. The cumulus mass and oocyte separate from the follicle wall, a process mediated by FSH; and they then float freely in the follicular fluid.

Ovulation

The processes of follicular rupture and expulsion of the oocyte and cumulus are still not fully understood, but involve interactions between LH, progesterone, prostaglandins, and proteolytic enzymes, and probably contractions of smooth muscle (Speroff *et al.* 1989*b*).

The corpus luteum

The collapsed follicle now becomes the corpus luteum. It is yellow in colour as a result of the uptake of the yellow pigment lutein by the enlarged granulosa cells. These cells have become vacuolated, and continue to grow for three more days. Some of the cells of the theca may also undergo a process of luteinization.

Vascularization occurs as the capillaries grow through the granulosa and enter the cavity, which usually fills with blood. This vascularization reaches its maximum by the ninth post-ovulatory day. The function of the corpus luteum is to produce oestrogen and increasing amounts of progesterone, the peak production of which corresponds to the time of maximum vascularization.

The corpus luteum requires the presence of LH to continue to function (Vande Wiele *et al.* 1970); but, beyond a certain point, administration of LH will not prolong the life-span of the corpus luteum. Unless fertilization and continued growth of the embryo has occurred, corpus luteal function begins to wane by the ninth to the eleventh post-ovulatory day. The mechanism of luteolysis in the human is not fully understood, but it is an active process, possibly mediated by intra-ovarian oestrogen or prostaglandins (Auletta and Flint 1988).

Intra-ovarian progesterone levels inhibit folliculogenesis. As the corpus luteum regresses, a fresh cohort of follicles escapes from this inhibition and begins to mature. The process of follicular development precedes the onset of the menses, which is the inevitable result of complete cessation of corpus luteum function.

In summary, the major follicular products during the ovarian cycle are:

1. (a) oestrogen until the immediately pre-ovulatory period and in the post-ovulatory phase; and

(b) progesterone in small quantities pre-ovulatorily, increasing to
   a maximum and then declining from the mid-luteal phase; and
2. the mature oocyte, which has completed the first meiotic division.

Hypothalamic and pituitary events

The hypothalamus and the pituitary lie at the base of the brain. The
major reproductive areas of the hypothalamus, the median eminence
and the arcuate nucleus, lie in close relationship to the third ventricle.
The pituitary, lying in the sella turcica of the skull, is connected to the
base of the brain by the pituitary stalk. There are no direct neuronal
connections between the hypothalamus and pituitary. Chemical
messages are relayed from one to the other (primarily from the
hypothalamus to the pituitary) by the portal system, a rich network
of capillaries which flows through the stalk (Everett 1969). There
may be a second system of communication by means of the cerebro-
spinal fluid of the third ventricle.

The anterior lobe of the pituitary is responsible for the synthesis,
storage, and release of a number of trophic hormones. Those
specifically involved in the reproductive process are FSH, LH, and
prolactin (PRL). The synchronization of follicular development,
ovulation, corpus luteum formation, and steroid hormone production
is modulated by the effects of LH and FSH. These pituitary hormones
are under the influence of gonadotrophin-releasing hormone
(GnRH), which is synthesized in the hypothalamus. The metabolism of GnRH is controlled by a number of neurotransmitters from
higher areas of the brain, and the whole system is driven by the
steroids produced by the ovary (Speroff *et al.* 1989*a*). Certain principles will be described to facilitate understanding of the interaction
of follicular and hypothalamic pituitary events through feedback
loops (Everett 1969).

Feedback loops

Simply stated, a feedback loop is a system whereby secretion of a
hormone exerts an effect upon its own production, either by influencing those signals controlling its production, or by influencing
directly the cells responsible for its production (Knobil 1980). A

direct effect of oestrogen upon its own production by the granulosa cells is an example of ultrashort-loop feedback; an effect of oestrogen upon the hypothalamic and pituitary metabolism of GnRH, LH, or FSH (Chappel *et al*. 1981), of long-loop feedback; and the effect of LH and FSH on the hypothalamic metabolism of GnRH, of short-loop feedback. Feedback effects may be negative or positive: thus the recognized effect of early-follicular-phase levels of oestrogen in reducing the pituitary responses to GnRH, and hence the release of LH and FSH, is negative long-loop feedback. Escape from this negative feedback control when oestrogen levels are very low after the menopause accounts for the very high levels of circulating gonadotrophins at that time (Sherman *et al*. 1976). The gonadotrophins can reduce the secretion of GnRH, an example of short-loop negative feedback.

When oestrogen levels increase in the follicular fluid, they directly increase the number of FSH receptors, thus increasing the production of oestrogen by the granulosa cells, an example of ultrashort-loop positive feedback (Richards 1980). The most striking example of positive feedback is the impact of high sustained levels of oestrogen at mid-cycle. Positive long-loop feedback acting at the pituitary produces the mid-cycle surge of LH (Menon *et al*. 1985).

The physiology of GnRH and the gonadotrophins

The hypothalamus responds to blood-borne and direct signals by the release of GnRH in a pulsatile fashion (Knobil 1980). GnRH is a decapeptide with a half life of two to four minutes.

The release of GnRH into the portal system is modified by:

1. *Neurotransmitters*: changes in the frequency and amplitude of the pulses of GnRH are

   - stimulated by centrally produced nor-epinephrine,

   - inhibited by dopamine, serotonin, and endorphins.

2. *The sex steroids*:

   - the negative feedback effect of the sex steroids is probably due to their ability to increase endorphin secretion, and hence the inhibition of GnRH metabolism.

3. A *direct short-loop feedback of the gonadotrophins*, exerting an in-hibitory effect (Speroff *et al.* 1989*a*).

The gonadotrophins are released from the pituitary in a pulsatile fashion which varies through the cycle. This release is modified by:

1. GnRH
   - GnRH stimulates synthesis, storage, and release of the gona-dotrophins.
2. Oestrogen and progesterone:
   - The effects of GnRH on the pituitary are modulated in the pituitary by local concentrations of the sex steroids. Low levels of oestrogen stimulate its synthetic and storage actions. These low levels do not effect the release of LH, but inhibit the release of FSH.
   - As oestrogen levels rise, the amounts of LH and FSH stored increase. When the critical levels of oestrogen have been attained and sustained at mid-cycle, the effects within the pituitary change from inhibitory to stimulatory (positive feed-back), with a resultant release of LH—the mid-cycle LH surge.
   - Progesterone at low levels acting in the pituitary increases secretion of LH and stimulates the mid-cycle surge of FSH. At high levels, progesterone inhibits GnRH metabolism in the hypothalamus and the ability of GnRH to stimulate gonado-trophin synthesis in and release from the pituitary.
3. Inhibin:
   - Inhibin is a peptide secreted by the granulosa in response to FSH. Inhibin suppresses the release of FSH from the pituitary.

Prolactin

Prolactin is the other important reproductive hormone produced by the anterior pituitary, and its primary function is to promote lacta-tion. In the non-pregnant adult, prolactin synthesis and storage are enhanced by a direct effect of oestrogen on the prolactin-secreting cells of the anterior pituitary—the lactotrophs. Secretion is tonically inhibited by dopamine, secreted by the hypothalamus into the portal system (Ben-Jonathan 1985).

The interaction between hypothalamic/pituitary and follicular function

The investigation and management of a woman's ovulatory status are dependent upon a clear understanding of the normal physiology. The preceding sections have considered the basic phenomena which occur in the ovary, hypothalamus, and pituitary. This section will describe the synchronous interrelationship of these events.

At the end of the luteal phase, corpus luteum function (oestrogen and progesterone production) wanes. Released from progesterone inhibition, a cohort of follicles begins to ripen. By removal of the negative-feedback effect of progesterone, FSH levels begin to rise. Menstruation occurs, and the gradually rising FSH levels stimulate follicular development and oestrogen production by the pre-antral follicles. Fluid accumulation transforms the pre-antral to the antral follicles, one of which gains dominance by the fifth day of the cycle. The negative-feedback effects of oestrogen and inhibin reduce FSH secretion. The effect of oestrogen on LH is mildly positive, and is reflected by a slight rise in the serum levels. By the ninth day, the dominant follicle is larger and more vascular. FSH in conjunction with oestrogen has induced LH receptors on follicular membranes. Circulating levels of oestrogen continue to rise, increasing the volume of gonadotrophins stored within the pituitary by sensitizing it to the production and storage effects of GnRH.

Under the influence of LH the pre-ovulatory follicle begins to luteinize and to produce progesterone, which exerts a positive-feedback effect on FSH production. This begins on the tenth day of the cycle. In the immediately pre-ovulatory period, oestrogen levels climb rapidly, exerting a positive-feedback effect on the pituitary which signals the start of the LH surge. The small rise in progesterone also triggers the mid-cycle FSH surge.

Within the ovary, the oocyte has completed the first meiotic division and is surrounded by the cumulus and lying free within the follicular fluid, an FSH-mediated event. About 12 hours after peak LH production, or 24 to 36 hours after the start of the LH surge, ovulation occurs and the corpus luteum is formed. There is a precipitate drop in oestrogen production which corresponds with the LH peak. Whether this represents a central or an ovarian event is unclear.

Progesterone production by the corpus luteum continues to rise, reaching a peak by the seventh post-ovulatory day. During this time, oestrogen production again increases. The negative-feedback effect of the steroids inhibits gonadotrophin secretion to levels which are lower than those of the follicular phase, although sufficient LH is produced to maintain the function of the corpus luteum.

Endometrial preparation for implantation

The events in the ovary have served to produce a mature oocyte and a series of steroid hormones. One effect of these hormones is to prepare the endometrium to accept the implantation of the embryo. These endometrial changes will now be described.

The uterine lining, with the exception of the basal layer, in which reside the bases of the endometrial glands, is shed during menstruation. The endometrium itself is composed of three major structures— the glands, the stroma, and the blood-vessels. The effect of oestrogen, elaborated by the follicle, is reparative following menstruation. The follicular phase of the ovarian cycle corresponds to the proliferative phase of the endometrial cycle. During the proliferative phase, the endometrium increases in thickness, the glands which are straight become longer, and their epithelium becomes columnar.

As the proliferative phase progresses, the stroma becomes more vascular, and the glands and vessels become coiled. Subnuclear aggregates of glycogen appear in the glandular cells. Following ovulation, and under the influence of oestrogen and progesterone during the luteal phase of the ovarian cycle, there is further thickening of the endometrium. As vascularization increases, the glands, which by now have become very convoluted, accumulate secretions, and the stroma becomes oedematous. This is the secretory phase of the endometrial cycle. More details of these changes are described later in this chapter, as they are particularly relevant to dating the endometrium.

In the final phase of the cycle, as oestrogen and progesterone levels wane, glandular activity wanes. The stroma is invaded by leukocytes. The spiral arterioles begin to constrict rhythmically, leading to ischaemic necrosis of their walls, through which blood begins to seep. Bleeding and sloughing of the endometrium heralds the onset of menstruation (Edwards 1980).

INVESTIGATION OF OVULATION

The physician investigating ovulation may wish to answer three questions:

1. Can the occurrence of ovulation be detected?
2. What is the quality of the ovulatory process?
3. Can the timing of ovulation be predicted?

The detection of ovulation

The release of the oocyte is an all-or-nothing phenomenon which can only be confirmed absolutely by the occurrence of pregnancy. Although follicular rupture *has* been observed ultrasonographically (O'Herlihy *et al.* 1980), this was a chance event, and cannot be relied upon in clinical practice.

All other tests are inferential, and are based upon:

(a) the menstrual history;
(b) direct hormone measurements;
(c) assessment of end organ changes produced by the steroid hormones; and
(d) ultrasonographic visualization of follicular development, disappearance of the dominant follicle, and formation of the corpus luteum.

The purpose of any test is to determine reliably whether or not a given event is occurring. As pregnancy, the gold standard, is an infrequent event, inferential tests must be measured one against the other. Thus the value of the menstrual history as a diagnostic test may be compared with direct measurements of luteal phase progesterone or the results of endometrial biopsy.

A clinically useful test should accurately indicate the occurrence (normal test) or non-occurrence (abnormal test) of an event, in this case ovulation. A very useful comparison between tests is the Kappa statistic, which measures agreement between two indicators (Fleiss 1981). Kappa values less than 0.40 indicate poor, between 0.40 and 0.75 good, and greater than 0.75 excellent agreement. Thus if serum progesterone values were elevated in 99 per cent of women with 28-day cycles, the Kappa value for the agreement between progesterone estimation and cycle history as diagnostic tests would exceed 0.75.

As well as being scientifically accurate, any clinical test should be as inexpensive and as non-invasive as possible, and consume as little of the patient's time as possible. With these criteria in mind, the various tests of the occurrence of ovulation will be discussed.

The menstrual history

The menstrual history will either be regular (21 to 35 days), reveal the absence of menses (no bleeding for three times the normal menstrual interval), or lie somewhere in between these two extremes.

Ninety-one to 97 per cent of women with a regular cycle (normal test result) have objective evidence of progesterone production (Rosenfeld and Garcia 1976; Orrell *et al.* 1980).

Absence of menses (amenorrhoea) occurs when there is anovulation, when the uterus cannot respond to the hormonal stimuli, or when there is occlusion of the cervix or within the vagina.

Irregular cycles (abnormal test result) do not reliably predict anovulation, as progesterone production may be present in 73 to 76 per cent of such cycles (Collins 1990*a*).

Thus obtaining a history of a regular cycle is an accurate, cheap, non-invasive, and convenient method of inferring that ovulation is occurring. Irregularity is insufficiently accurate to confirm anovulation.

Direct hormonal measurements

Application of the knowledge of the physiological events described earlier in this chapter would imply that the pre-ovulatory LH surge or the luteal production of progesterone could serve as indicators that ovulation was imminent or had occurred.

LH surge

The mid-cycle LH surge can be detected by serial blood or urine sampling and laboratory analysis by either radio-immuno-assay (RIA) or enzyme-linked immuno-sorbent assay (ELISA). Commercial kits are available for home urine testing. While these avenues may be helpful to time ovulation, they are of little value simply to detect ovulation, particularly in women with irregular cycles, requiring as they do repeated daily measurements. They are no more accurate than the menstrual history in the regularly menstruating woman, but are much more expensive and time-consuming.

Luteal production of progesterone

An increase in progesterone values, or those of its metabolites in blood, urine, and saliva, are generally accepted as evidence of ovulation. Sampling with the peripheral blood is usually performed. Twenty-four hour urine samples are required to estimate levels of the progesterone metabolite, pregnanediol. Salivary progesterone values will be about 1 per cent of those in plasma, but correlate reasonably well with peripheral blood concentrations (Riad-Fahmy *et al*. 1987).

What level of progesterone should be accepted as evidence of ovulation? Even with a low cutpoint (10 nmol/l) secretory endometrium is found in 42 per cent of so-called cases of anovulation (Table 3.1) (Rosenfeld and Garcia 1976). When the cutpoint is raised to 39 nmol/l, progesterone values below this cutpoint are associated with secretory endometrium in 90 per cent of cases. The Kappa statistic is an estimate of the agreement beyond that due to chance; at this cutpoint the Kappa value is 0.14, indicating that the observed agreement is mainly due to chance. The cutpoint giving the best agreement (Kappa = 0.79) was 16 nmol/l (Abdulla *et al*. 1983).

The measurement of progesterone should be made in the mid-luteal phase. Sampling in the morning reduces the impact of the recognized fluctuations of progesterone levels in response to variations in LH production (Filicori *et al*. 1984).

Single mid-luteal progesterone estimates in regularly menstruating women, or weekly sampling from day 21 in women with

Table 3.1 *Frequency of secretory endometrium associated with various cutpoints in plasma progesterone concentration*

Progesterone cutpoint (nmol/l)	Frequency of secretory endometrium (per cent, 95 per cent confidence limits)		Kappa value	No. of subjects
	Normal progesterone result	Abnormal progesterone result		
10	98 (96,100)	42 (23,61)	0.63	234*
16	100	33 (0,86)	0.79	72†
30	100	82 (59,100)	0.27	72†
39	100	90 (77,100)	0.14	72†

* Rosenfeld and Garcia 1976
† Abdulla *et al.* 1983

irregular cycles, are sufficient to confirm the presumptive occurrence of ovulation if values equal or exceed 16 nmol/l.

Assessment of end organ changes

Changes dependent upon oestrogen production include:

1. Peri-ovulatory changes in salivary electrical resistance and electrical impedance across the vaginal mucosa (Albrecht *et al.* 1985), which are no more accurate than the menstrual history (Collins 1990*a*).

2. Changes in cervical mucus, from fluid in the predominantly oestrogenic pre-ovulatory phase to sticky in the post-ovulatory progesterone phase, are insufficiently accurate to confirm that ovulation has occurred.

Changes dependent upon progesterone production

The basal body-temperature graph

Progesterone will raise the basal body-temperature (BBT) by 0.2 °C. The patient is instructed to record her temperature, orally, rectally, or vaginally, using the basal thermometer immediately upon wakening and before getting out of bed. The results are plotted on a chart.

Three consecutive values should be 0.2 °C higher than the preceding 6 values, and these changes should occur within a period of 48 hours or less to be regarded as presumptive evidence that ovulation has occurred (WHO 1983).

While it is a cheap and non-invasive test, the BBT leaves a certain amount to be desired. Monophasic patterns can occur in from 11 per cent (Orrell *et al*. 1980) to 75 per cent (Moghissi 1976*a*) of cycles subsequently determined to have been ovulatory. The BBT is no more accurate than the history as a method of detecting ovulation. Its only value is one of convenience for the patient who is unable to attend on the appropriate mid-luteal day for venepuncture to obtain samples for progesterone measurement.

Endometrial biopsy

The endometrial biopsy allows the histological identification of progesterone-mediated changes which historically have been accepted as presumptive evidence of ovulation (Noyes *et al*. 1950). The test is painful, inconvenient, and adds little to the information gained from the combination of the menstrual history and serum progesterone values if simple confirmation of ovulation is all that is required. Its role in assessing the quality of ovulation will be discussed later.

Ultrasound methods

Hackeloer (1978), using ultrasound scanning, first followed the developing follicles in normal menstrual cycles. Sequential daily scanning is able to detect the gradual growth of the follicle and its transformation to a corpus luteum in 90 per cent of cycles studied (Queenan *et al*. 1980). This method is too expensive and time-consuming to be used in routine practice simply to confirm ovulation.

Summary

The proportion of cycles that are ovulatory, as predicted by various index tests compared with standard criteria, is shown in Table 3.2. Of the various methods available to detect ovulation, attention to the menstrual history and the estimation of mid-luteal serum pro-

Table 3.2 *Detection of ovulation by cycle history or basal temperature compared with endometrial biopsy or serum progesterone estimation*

Cycles	Percentage of cycles shown to be ovulatory by endometrial biopsy or serum progesterone estimation (95 per cent CI)*		Kappa value	Subjects Number	Authors
	Regular	Irregular			
	96 (93,99)	76 (61,91)	0.25	218	Rosenfeld and Garcia 1976
	97 (94,100)	74 (57,91)	0.29	200	Orrell *et al.* 1980
Basal temperature	Biphasic	Monophasic			
	100	75 (45,100)	0.33	29	Moghissi 1976*a*
	97 (95,99)	11 (0,32)	0.71	200	Orrell *et al.* 1980
	98 (93,100)	0	0.79	44	Magyar *et al.* 1979

* As determined by endometrial biopsy or serum progesterone estimation

gesterone are the simplest, most accurate, least invasive, and least expensive.

Evaluation of the quality of ovulation

While ovulation is clearly an all-or-nothing phenomenon, it has been suggested that subtle defects in this process may cause infertility. If such is the case, it would seem reasonable to insist that such phenomena would occur repeatedly in the same individual, that their prevalence would be greater in an infertile than a fertile population, and that randomized studies of treatment versus no treatment would show a distinct improvement in the pregnancy rate in the treated group. Two such postulated defects, luteinized unruptured follicle syndrome (LUFS), and luteal phase defect (LPD), require consideration.

The luteinized unruptured follicle syndrome was described when no evidence of an ovulation stigma could be seen on the corpus luteum at the time of laparoscopy (Marik and Hulka 1978; Koninckx *et al.* 1978). They argued that, although the appropriate hormonal changes had occurred, the oocyte had not been released. Subsequently, it has been shown that, if normal mid-luteal progesterone levels reflected normal follicular development, then ultrasound scanning rarely revealed failure of follicular rupture (Coutts *et al.* 1982). This syndrome has yet to be shown to be a consistent finding in the same patient, nor is the prevalence in the fertile population known. Until the status of LUFS is clarified, it should not be sought as part of the routine evaluation.

It has also been suggested that, although the oocyte may be released, there may be a relative deficiency of progesterone effect upon the endometrium: the luteal phase defect (LPD) (Jones 1949). It is worth quoting Wentz (1990) 'The condition has never been shown to be the *cause* of infertility in a great percentage of patients . . . nor has it . . . been possible to demonstrate that these patients have benefited from the standpoint of pregnancy initiation and outcome'.

Undoubtedly, blastocyst attachment and function depend upon normal function of the corpus luteum (Andrews 1979; Wentz 1980). The production of progesterone by the corpus luteum is at least in part responsible for maturation of the endometrium. Assessment of the quality of ovulation has concentrated upon clinical assessment of the duration of the luteal phase, histological assessment of the endometrium, and measurement of serum progesterone levels.

Length of the luteal phase

The time from ovulation to the onset of the menses is usually more consistent than the pre-ovulatory period. Even so, Lenton *et al.* (1984) have demonstrated that, in normal women, the 95 per cent confidence interval for the length of the luteal phase is 10 to 17 days. Even a documented duration of less than 11 days is not a clinically useful test for the diagnosis of LPD (Lenton *et al.* 1984; Landgren *et al.* 1980). The elevation of basal body temperature lasts for less than 11 days in 18 per cent of apparently normal women (Marshall 1963).

Histological examination

In the classic study of endometrial histological changes by Noyes *et al.* (1950), ovulation was assumed to occur on day 14. By cycle day 18, the size of the subnuclear vacuoles of the glandular cells was diminished. Concurrently, acidophilic intraluminary secretions had begun to appear. 'The behaviour of the glandular epithelium has been the key to dating the first half of the secretory phase.' By day 23, stromal changes were more marked, the spiral arterioles were more prominent, and mitotic changes were noticeable in the peri-arteriolar stromal cells. Noyes *et al.* (1950) described the findings as 'pre-decidual' changes.

By cycle day 24, definite collections of these pre-decidual cells were easily identifiable, and stromal mitoses were evident. Islands of pre-decidual cells had begun to appear just below the surface epithelium by day 25, and had coalesced to form a continuous sheet by day 27. One event, when taken in conjunction with these stromal changes, served to identify the twenty-sixth day. No polymorphonuclear leukocytes were visible on day 25; but an invasion by these cells began on day 26, and was characteristic by day 27. The twenty-sixth day, therefore, was specifically identified by the presence of polymorphonuclear leukocytes and islands of predecidual cells which had not yet coalesced to form a continuous subepithelial sheet.

When Noyes *et al.* (1950) analysed these histological findings, they were not accurate in predicting the date of subsequent menstruation. Of 300 patients studied, 42 (14 per cent) menstruated on the day predicted, 36 (12 per cent) menstruated later, and 222 (74 per cent) menstruated earlier. The authors concluded that the biopsy was a better marker for the progestational effect, rather than for predicting the time of onset of the next menstrual period. It is for this reason that the day upon which the biopsy is taken (ideally, day 26) is calculated by assigning the first day of the next period as day 28 (irrespective of the length of the cycle) and subtracting from this the number of days between the biopsy procedure and the onset of menses. A diagnosis of LPD is made if the dated biopsy is reported as being two or more days out of phase with the calculated date at which it was taken, in two or more cycles. Recent publications permit a reappraisal of these original observations.

Errors could potentially occur from either biological variability within and between individuals, or from observer inaccuracy. Intra-observer error occurs in observations made by one observer, and inter-observor error occurs when two observers interpret the same object.

To reduce the effects of biological variability, late rather than mid-luteal biopsies appear to be more consistent (Kusuda *et al.* 1983). However, biological variations are still common in a single individual, making interpretation difficult (Li *et al.* 1989). Most studies used the onset of the next menstrual period to determine the chronological date.

If, instead, the LH peak is used as the fixed point from which the chronological date is measured, accuracy improves (Li *et al.* 1987). Among thirteen parous volunteers, for example, the histological changes were assessed independently by two observers, and the chronological date set by ultrasound assessment of follicular rupture, serum LH measurement, temperature graphing, and the onset of the next menstrual period (Shoupe *et al.* 1989). When the date of ovulation was fixed by ultrasound the histological dating was within 2 days in 25 to 26 interpretations (96 per cent), but when the histological findings were compared with the onset of the next period, only 17 to 26 (65 per cent) were congruent.

Intra-observer error was assessed in a study of 63 samples dated independently by the same observer on two occasions. Disagreement of more than two days (intra-observer error) occurred in 10 per cent (Li *et al.* 1989). Inter-observer error was evaluated in a study of 62 specimens by 5 pathologists (Scott *et al.* 1988); the mean inter-observer variability in dating specimens was nearly 1 day (0.96, SE 0.08)—a variability which was affected by neither the endometrial maturity nor the presence of maturation delay.

When both biological variability and the potential for both intra- and inter-observer error are taken into account, it is clear that histological dating of the endometrium is, at best, an unreliable indicator of the endometrial response to progesterone. It logically follows that the use of this technique to diagnose the luteal phase defect is inaccurate.

Using the criterion of 2 or more days out-of-phase, 4 to 27 per cent of biopsies were judged to be abnormal among fertile women (Balasch *et al.* 1986; Davis *et al.* 1989). The frequency of endometrial retardation was 2 to 45 per cent in collected series of women complaining of infertility (Annos *et al.* 1980; Huang 1986; Moszkowski *et al.* 1962; Pittaway *et al.* 1983; Rosenberg *et al.* 1980; Wentz 1980). Li *et al.* (1991) found that endometrial development was more than two days retarded in significantly more women with unexplained infertility (mean duration six years) than either fertile women or in those with tubal factor infertility. The search for a link with fertility should, perhaps, be conducted among women with such prolonged and otherwise unexplained infatility.

Although the repeated occurrence of LPD would be needed to show that it caused infertility, studies on repeated biopsies are subject to bias. Women in whom the first biopsy is normal are often unwilling to undergo a repeat procedure. Thus, women with abnormal first biopsy reports form an excessively large proportion of the subjects in studies of repeated endometrial biopsy results. Also, if the results of the first biopsy are not blinded, observer bias is inevitable. Even so, the reported agreement between first and second biopsy results is little better than would be expected by chance, as shown by the Kappa values in Table 3.3 (Kappa values < 0.40 = poor agreement; 0.40 to 0.75 = good agreement).

When three biopsies are obtained, only 4 per cent are normal

Table 3.3 *Correlation between the results of first and second endometrial biopsy reports*

| Number of subjects | Percentage of second biopsy results reported as LPD (95 per cent CI)* | | Kappa value | Authors |
	First biopsy normal	First biopsy abnormal		
300	20 (13,27)	52 (45,59)	0.30	Balasch *et al*. 1985
81	17 (7,27)	48 (29,67)	0.33	Kusuda *et al*. 1983
39	36 (8,64)	79 (64,94)	0.40	Wentz 1980
21	47 (23,67)	25 (0,67)	−0.15	Driessen *et al*. 1980

* LPD, luteal phase defect; CI, confidence interval

when the first and second biopsies have been consistently out-of-phase (Balasch *et al*. 1985). Even among such women, however, successful pregnancy has been reported without treatment (Balasch *et al*. 1986).

Much more meticulous work is required before a clear clinical interpretation can be attached to the results of the endometrial biopsy. Given that the biopsy is painful and time-consuming, and given our present state of understanding, of little clinical value, assessment of serum progesterone levels might offer an attractive alternative means of evaluating luteal function.

Endocrine assessment

There is still no single definition for luteal phase adequacy based on progesterone concentration (Collins 1990*a*). Assessment of the pattern of progesterone secretion would require daily sampling, which is obviously impractical. To address this difficulty, clinical investigators have employed either a limited number of repeated samples or single estimations.

In one study based on repeated sampling, the sum of three mid-luteal progesterone values was never less than 48 nmol/l in apparently normal patients (Abraham *et al*. 1974). In another Landgren *et al* (1980) demonstrated a sustained progesterone concentration above 16 nmol/l in 94 per cent of volunteers with regular cycles. In studies based on single mid-luteal values, the cutpoints used to determine normality ranged from 20 to 40 nmol/l (Abdulla *et al.* 1983; Hull *et al.* 1982*a*). Even these values leave a certain amount to be desired. If a cutpoint of 20 nmol/l is taken, 20 per cent of normal women would be classified as suffering from progesterone deficiency (Wathen *et al.* 1984).

The reported criteria for progesterone values are summarized in Table 3.4. The proportion of cases judged to be abnormal based on cut-points in the 15 to 45 nmol/l range varied from 6 per cent to 70 per cent, and the data revealed no correlation between cutpoint value and the frequency of abnormal results (Goldstein *et al.* 1982; Radwanska *et al.* 1981; Rosenfeld *et al.* 1980; Shangold *et al.* 1983; Shepard and Senturia 1977; Zorn *et al.* 1984).

Glazener *et al.* (1988) compared mid-luteal progesterone values in 579 cycles in 159 women complaining of unexplained infertility with 267 cycles among 58 normal women. There were no significant differences in the mean progesterone values or in the incidence of

Table 3.4 *Reported criteria for adequate luteal function based on progesterone concentrations in peripheral blood samples*

Progesterone cutpoint (nmol/l)	Description	Authors
Repeated sampling		
48	Lowest sum of three mid-luteal values among volunteers in cycles with an LH peak and luteal phase more than 12 days*	Abraham *et al.* 1974
16	In volunteers with cycles 26–35 days, 94 per cent had sustained elevation of progesterone over 16 nmol/l for 5 days	Landgren *et al.* 1980
Single mid-luteal values		
20	20th percentile of values in ovulatory cycles among volunteers	Wathen *et al.* 1984
30	10th percentile of values in cycles of conception among infertile women	Hull *et al.* 1982*a*
40	20th percentile of values in cycles of conception among infertile women	Abdulla *et al.* 1983

* LH: Luteinizing hormone

cycles with progesterone values of less than 20 nmol/l (17 per cent versus 15 per cent) in the 2 groups respectively. Even when the cutpoint was dropped to 14 nmol/l, the frequency of abnormal values was similar in the comparison groups (4 per cent vs 3 per cent). Because cycles with low values of progesterone may occur as a random phenomenon in both fertile and infertile women, these authors concluded that 'luteal defect . . . in women with normal menstrual cycles must be a rare entity and requires at least six cycles of investigation (*or none*)' (author's italics).

It is possible that a luteal defect exists only when abnormal histological dating and abnormally low progesterone values co-incide. In some studies, abnormal progesterone values are slightly more likely to be correlated with an abnormal biopsy result (Annos *et al.* 1980; Balasch *et al.* 1985; Goldstein *et al.* 1982; Rosenfeld *et al.* 1983; Shangold *et al.* 1983; Shepard and Senturia 1977; Zorn *et al.* 1984), but only two of seven studies reported a significant cor-relation between histological and hormonal values (Goldstein *et al.* 1982; Zorn *et al.* 1984). The weighted Kappa statistic for the 7 studies was 0.18, suggesting that the overall agreement is little better than the agreement expected from chance alone (Collins 1990*a*). Li *et al.* (1991) found that progesterone profiles, even among women with retarded endometrial development, were not different from those of fertile women.

It must be concluded that the usefulness of histological dating and measurements of the serum progesterone values as presently understood contribute little to the understanding of the cause of otherwise unexplained infertility. This is particularly so when it is recognized that pregnancy occurs with similar frequency in women with normal endometrium and in women with delayed endometrial development (Balasch *et al.* 1986).

It also has been suggested that minor aberrations in the metab-olism of prolactin, insufficient to cause anovulation, may interfere with normal luteal function (Balasch and Vanrell 1987). A possible mechanism could exist, as prolactin can be shown to inhibit pro-gesterone production by luteal cells *in vitro* (McNatty *et al.* 1974). Nevertheless, there is no correlation between prolactin levels and progesterone concentration or conception (Glazener *et al.* 1987*a*; Sarris *et al.* 1978). Also, controlled studies of treatment with bromocriptine (Glazener *et al.* 1987*b*; McBain and Pepperell 1982; Wright *et al.* 1979) have failed to demonstrate any improvement in pregnancy rates. Glazener *et al.* (1987*a*) conclude that in women with normal menstrual cycles it is generally not worth measuring prolactin.

With our present state of understanding, ovulatory status is best evaluated by taking a good cycle history, supplemented by the mid-luteal measurement of serum progesterone. Anovulation is a cause of infertility.

If ovulation is occurring on a regular basis, further investigation is unlikely to reveal an explanation for the patient's inability to conceive. Attention will now be directed towards predicting the time of ovulation.

Prediction of the timing of ovulation

It has long been believed that if the time of ovulation could be predicted accurately, couples could be advised about the best time to have intercourse, to improve their chances of spontaneous pregnancy. This section will examine the methods currently available to predict the day of ovulation. How these methods do or do not achieve better fertility will be discussed.

Methods

The following techniques have been applied in attempts to predict ovulation:

(1) clinical information;

(2) basal body temperature graphing

(3) end-organ response;

(4) estimations of hormone concentrations; and

(5) ultrasound imaging.

Clinical information

McIntosh *et al.* (1980) evaluated 293 cycles in 88 normally men-struating women. The data derived from these observations permitted calculation of the precise day of ovulation to within 95 per cent confidence. This procedure is only of value in women with regular (28–29 day) cycles. In an individual woman, if the cycles over the preceding 8 months range from 26 to 34 days, the 95 per cent confidence interval of the predicted follicular phase-length in the next cycle is 12 to 19 days, which clearly is not sufficiently accurate.

Basal body temperature (BBT) graphing

The lowest point of BBT immediately preceding the post-ovulatory rise, the nadir, has been used to predict ovulation. The range of correct predictions is shown in Table 3.5, with accuracies ranging from 5 to 85 per cent. This method is somewhat less than infallible.

End-organ response

1. Cervical mucus sampling daily in the peri-ovulatory period may permit a degree of accuracy of prediction of 80 per cent (Vermesh *et al.* 1987). In three reported groups (Table 3.5), the range was from 56 to 80 per cent. If the test is to be performed by a physician or nurse, several daily attendances are required, at considerable inconvenience to the patient.
2. Vaginal electrical impedance has a range of accuracy of prediction of 33 to 59 per cent (Albrecht *et al.* 1985). The method can be performed by the patient. Further reports must be awaited to validate this procedure.

Estimations of hormone concentrations

Laboratory detection of the beginning of the LH surge

Ovulation will occur 24 to 36 hours after the start of the LH surge. Detection of the rise of LH values requires multiple daily venepunctures or urine collections. These are expensive and time-consuming.

Home ovulation prediction kits

These are dependent upon detection in urine of the LH surge, and can be used by the patient. They are expensive, and can be affected

Table 3.5 *Methods for predicting the day of ovulation compared with luteinizing hormone or ultrasound evaluation*

Diagnostic test	Definition of ovulation*	Correct predictions per cent (95 per cent CI)	Number in study	Authors
BBT nadir				
	US	5 (0,13)	15	Fedele *et al.* 1988
	LH	85 (73,97)	66	Garcia *et al.* 1981
	LH	55 (42,68)	47	Lenton *et al.* 1977
	LH	63 (49,77)	27	Morris *et al.* 1976
	LH	47 (36,58)	60	Quagliarello and Arny 1986
	US	29 (10,39)	28	Vermesh *et al.* 1987
Cervical mucus				
	US	59 (32,86)	15	Fedele *et al.* 1988
	LH	56 (44,68)	63	Garcia *et al.* 1981
	US	80 (66,94)	49	Leader *et al.* 1985
Self-test LH kits				
	LH	100 (83,100)	24	Elkind-Hirsch *et al.* 1986
	US	64 (50,77)	15	Garcia *et al.* 1981
	LH	100 (82,100)	16	Knee *et al.* 1985
	LH	90 (72,100)	10	Martinez *et al.* 1986
	US	53 (40,66)	30	Vermesh *et al.* 1987

* LH: lutenizing hormone peak ±24 hours; US: disappearance of dominant follicle; BBT: basal body temperature

by ambient temperature (Roberts and Braude 1987). The range of correct prediction is from 53 to 100 per cent (Table 3.5). The higher levels of accuracy occurred in studies which compared urinary LH kits with LH detection in the serum. Lower levels of correlation were noted when the kits were compared with ultrasonographic detection of disappearance of the dominant follicle (Fedele *et al.* 1988).

The ultimate criterion by which any procedure used in infertility should be judged is whether or not it improves pregnancy rates. Donor insemination programmes, which depend upon accurate prediction of ovulation, provide excellent models for comparison of timing methods.

When the accuracy and predictive values of serum and urinary hormone tests, vaginal impedance, cervical mucus, and peak values of urinary LH and oestradiol were compared, it was concluded that ovulation should be predicted by identification of the LH peak (Grinstead *et al.* 1989).

Table 3.6 shows the fecundability rates when LH kits were compared with standard methods such as BBT, cycle averaging, and cervical mucus assessment (Barratt *et al.* 1989*a*; Kossoy *et al.* 1988; Odem *et al.* 1991). The retrospective cohort study of Kossoy *et al.* (1988) involved women who received fresh donor semen for 7 to 16 months. Barratt *et al.* (1989*a*) randomly allocated women receiving donor insemination to the use of either urinary LH kits or BBT for six months. The increased fecundability with the LH kits in these studies was small and not significant. Odem *et al.* (1991) assigned women by hospital number to receive either two donor inseminations based on BBT or one insemination based on LH kit results

Table 3.6 *Evaluation of home self-tests of lutenizing hormone (LH) peaks for timing of donor insemination*

Authors	Fecundability per cycle		Number of women
	LH self-test	Standard timing	
Barratt *et al.* 1989*a*	0.07	0.04	53
Kossoy *et al.* 1988	0.13	0.11	120
Odem *et al.* 1991	0.06	0.13	113

during each of six cycles. The pregnancy rate was significantly higher ($p < 0.025$) and the cost was lower in the BBT group.

Ultrasound imaging

Disappearance of the dominant follicle detected ultrasonographically is the accepted gold standard for the timing of the occurrence of ovulation (Vermesh *et al.* 1987). Prediction is based upon the probable occurrence of ovulation 24 to 36 hours after the dominant follicle has attained a mean diameter of 2.2 cm. This technique is expensive and time-consuming.

Clinical applications

Timing of intercourse

To optimize their chances of spontaneous conception, couples are commonly advised to time intercourse, usually by using the BBT. The frequency of coitus is related to the probability of conception, rising from 15 per cent to 50 per cent in 6 months as the frequency of coitus rises from less than once per week to three times per week (MacLeod and Gold 1953). It is doubtful that aiming for the 'right day' irrespective of the method used, can improve upon these rates.

Further, there is a tendency among couples to 'save up' the ejaculate. This may improve the number of spermotozoa, but it may reduce their motility (Freund 1962). If the method of timing is inaccurate, then the resultant reduction of coital frequency theoretically could reduce the chances of conception. Insistence on a rigid protocol of sexual performance is one of the major stresses loaded upon these couples by well-meaning advisers.

On the other hand, many couples wish to feel that they are working on their own behalf and exerting some control over their destiny. They need not be deprived of the opportunity to use the BBT or urinary LH kits, provided they are given the accurate information that in most circumstances these manœuvres have not been shown to improve the pregnancy rates (Corsan *et al.* 1990).

CONCLUSIONS

If anovulation is detected, a cause for infertility has been established. From the evidence presented in this chapter, it is concluded that our ability accurately to assess the quality of ovulation is insufficiently well-developed to permit an explanation of infertility based on ovum retention in the luteinized follicle, a defective luteal phase, or minor variations in prolactin concentration. If ovulation is occurring, an event most simply confirmed by cycle history and mid-luteal progesterone estimation, then, with respect to the ovulatory process, the infertility is unexplained.

Definition

The first prerequisite to establish the diagnosis of unexplained infertility is the confirmation that ovulation is apparently occurring on a regular basis.

---

4 The production of spermotozoa and their transport in the male genital tract

PHYSIOLOGY

The production of spermatozoa begins at puberty and is continuous throughout the life-span of the male. For conception to occur, the spermatozoa initially must be transported from their site of origin to the cervix. While sperm production and sperm transport are different physiological events, clinical evaluation of both phenomena is performed by assessment of a fresh sample of the ejaculate. This section will describe:

1. the physiology of sperm production; and
2. the physiology of sperm transport in the male.

Physiology of sperm production

The events occurring within the testes and accessory glands, and within the hypothalamus and pituitary, and the interaction between the testes and these higher centres will be described.

Testicular and accessory gland events

Anatomy

The testes are paired ovoid organs which lie in the scrotum. They are 5 cm in length and have a volume of at least 20 ml. Each has an external coat, the tunica vaginalis, immediately below which lies the tunica albuginea. This latter is a dense, fibrous, non-distensible structure. On the postero-medical aspect of the testes the tunica albuginea invaginates to form the mediastinum testis, wherein lie the channels of the rete testis. Between the tunica albuginea and the rest of the testicular body is the tunica vasculosa, a layer of loose connective tissue containing many blood-vessels. A series of fibrous septa runs from the tunica albuginea to the mediastinum testis, dividing the organ into functional lobules. Each lobule contains between 250 and 400 seminiferous tubules. Each tubule is surrounded by Leydig cells (interstitial cells), which are responsible for testosterone secretion. The seminiferous tubules consist of a basement membrane upon which are situated sertoli cells and spermatogonia, which are the precursors for spermatogenesis. The seminiferous tubules are highly convoluted through the greater part of their length, becoming straight just before the testicular mediastinum. The straight portion is known as the tubulus rectus. These tubuli recti empty into the rete testis, from the upper pole of which 15 to 20 ducts, the efferent ductules, emerge. The ductules are surrounded by myoid cells.

The efferent ductules converge to form the epididymal duct, which has a length of six metres. It is lined with highly active epithelium, and is surrounded by smooth muscle. The entire epididymal duct is highly convoluted. The efferent ductules, the epididymal duct, and the proximal part of the vas deferens are known collectively as the epididymis, which lies on the postero-medial aspect of the testis. The epididymis has three identifiable sections, the upper being the caput, the middle portion the corpus, and the lower portion the cauda. The most distal portion of the cauda epididymis thickens considerably to form the muscular vas deferens, which is lined with ciliated columnar epithelium. The vas runs along the spermatic cord through the inguinal ring and into the abdominal cavity, crossing the ureter at its insertion to the bladder. Immediately behind the ureter lies the seminal vesicle, which is a tightly convoluted blind tube lined with mucus-secreting columnar epithelium. The duct of the seminal vesicle and the vas come together to form the ejaculatory duct. The paired ejaculatory ducts pass through the prostate between the medial and two lateral lobes to enter the urethra posteriorly through two slit-like orifices on the verumontanum of the prostate.

The prostate is an important accessory sex gland. It is enclosed in a muscular coat and made up of three lobes—two lateral and one median. A number of small ducts from the prostate enter the prostatic urethra in close conjunction with the ejaculatory orifices.

The urethra passes from the neck of the bladder, through the prostate, to the tip of the penis. Two small lobulated glands, the bulbo-urethral glands, open into the membranous urethra and secrete small amounts of mucus. At the distal end of the penile urethra urethral glands also contribute to mucus secretion.

Events in the testes and accessory glands

Testes

The testes serve two functions—the production of hormones and the production of spermatozoa. The two are closely interrelated, and are functions of the Leydig and sertoli cells and the germinal epithelium.

The Leydig cells are irregularly shaped, and lie within the loose connective tissue surrounding the seminiferous tubules. They are responsible, under the influence of pituitary LH, for testosterone production (Moudgal *et al*. 1971). Testosterone is responsible systemically for development and maintenance of the secondary sexual characteristics. It plays an integral role in spermatogenesis. Once produced by the Leydig cells, testosterone diffuses through the basement membrane into the sertoli cells. These are tall irregular cells lying on the basement membrane. Once the sertoli cells have been primed by the presence of FSH, most of their intracellular events can be maintained by testosterone. The major event is an increase in cyclic adenosine monophosphate (cAMP) production, resulting in the stimulation of a cAMP-dependent protein kinase (Dorrington *et al*. 1972). The kinase phosphorylates a number of sertoli cell proteins, the most important of which is the androgen-binding protein (ABP), which is secreted into the lumen of the seminiferous tubule (Hansson *et al*. 1973). In addition, the sertoli cells produce inhibin, which has a negative-feedback effect upon the pituitary production and release of FSH (Setchell and Jacks 1974).

The primitive germ cells arise in the yolk sac. By the third week of embryonic life, they have migrated to the gonadal ridge, and are described as gonocytes (Witschi 1948). By the third month, the primitive gonocytes have become transformed into spermatogonia.

The spermatogonia lie among the sertoli cells. Initially, they undergo mitotic division. Two types are recognizable; dark type A and pale type A. Both types differentiate into type B. Further mitoses transform the type B spermatogonia into primary spermatocytes. The first meiotic division occurs with the production of two secondary spermatocytes, which in turn give rise to four spermatids after the second meiotic step. This process from the spermatogonia to the haploid spermatid is called 'spermatogenesis' (Jequier 1986).

The spermatid is haploid and round-shaped. It will undergo four stages —golgi, cap, acrosome, and maturation—before it is recognizable as a spermatozoon. These steps are collectively referred to as 'spermiogenesis'. During these events, the cell has been moving away from the basement membrane towards the lumen of the tubule. The final intratesticular step whereby the spermatozoon separates from the sertoli cell is referred to as 'spermiation'.

The spermatozoa now move to the epididymis, where further maturation takes place. Changes occur in their structure, membranes, and ability to become fully motile. These changes are androgen-dependent.

Production of a mature spermatozoon from the spermatocyte takes about 80 to 100 days. Seventy days are required for the intratesticular events, and a further 20 to 30 days are required for epididymal maturation (Heller and Clairmont 1963). During this time, the cells are at risk of being exposed to various adverse influences, as will shortly be described. This occult life history of the sperm cell is but one of the factors which makes interpretation of the semen analysis so difficult.

Anatomy of the human sperm

The human sperm has a head, a mid-piece, and a tail. The head measures $4.5 \, \mu m \times 3 \, \mu m \times 1.5 \, \mu m$. It is composed mainly of the nucleus, which contains the haploid chromatin. The upper two-thirds are covered by the inner and outer acrosome membranes. The equatorial ridge divides the post-acrosomal lower third of the sperm head.

The mid-piece and tail together measure $50 \, \mu m$. From the head to the tip of the tail runs the axoneme. This structure is composed of nine paired and two single microtubules. In the mid-piece, the axoneme is surrounded by a helix of mitochondria. The outer portion of the mid-piece and all but the tip of the tail are encased in a fibrous sheath.

Accessory glands

The ejaculate is composed of spermatozoa and seminal plasma. The testes only account for 5 per cent of the total volume, with the remaining 95 per cent being contributed by the accessory glands (Lundquist 1949). The bulk of the ejaculate is derived from the seminal vesicles and the prostate.

A very small amount of fluid accompanies the spermatozoa from the rete testes to the caput epididymis. It is rich in testosterone, ABP, and inhibin. The epididymis actually absorbs water from the seminal fluid, and contributes inositol, carnitine, lipids, phospholipids, and epididymis motility protein (Brandt *et al.* 1978; Turner 1979).

Seminal vesicles   More than half of the total ejaculate comes from the seminal vesicles. Their contributions of fructose and prostaglandins are critical to sperm motility. From them is derived a fibrinogen-like substance which is responsible for immediate post-ejaculatory coagulation of the semen (Tauber and Zaneveld 1976).

Prostate   The prostate contributes 13 to 33 per cent of the ejaculate. An enzyme from the prostate acts upon the fibrinogen-like substance to effect coagulation. Prostatically-produced proteins liquefy the coagulum (Gotterer *et al.* 1955). Acid phosphatase, calcium, and zinc are all secreted by the prostate, as is spermine, a bacteriostatic amine (Karacagil *et al.* 1989).

Bulbo-urethral and urethral glands   The mucus of these glands, while small in volume, can be critically important. It is from these glands that anti-sperm antibodies may be secreted.

Hypothalamic and pituitary events

As in the female, the pituitary synthesizes, stores, and releases both the gonadotrophins, LH and FSH, and prolactin. The metabolism of the gonadotrophins is modified by GnRH. Prolactin is held under tonic inhibition.

Testosterone acts both at the hypothalamus, where it exhibits an acute inhibition of GnRH, and hence of LH release, and chronically at the level of the pituitary, thus maintaining daily testosterone output at a fairly constant level. Testosterone does not affect FSH metabolism.

Interactions between the testes and the higher centres

The spermatogonia mature to primary spermatocytes without any hormonal stimulus. Further maturation is dependent upon the presence of FSH and high local levels of testosterone.

FSH is required to initiate spermatogenesis at the time of puberty (Steinberger 1971). Unless it is present, LH exerts no effect. The primary function of FSH is to induce LH receptors on the Leydig cells. Once these receptors have been induced, LH promotes testosterone formation (Swerdloff *et al.* 1985). The Leydig cells also possess receptors for prolactin, physiological levels of which stimulate testosterone secretion, whereas elevated levels inhibit testosterone production;

FSH acts directly upon the sertoli cells to produce ABP (Steinberger *et al.* 1975). Testosterone is bound to the ABP, thus producing the high local levels of testosterone necessary for maturation of the primary spermatocyte to the young spermatid. The final maturation of the young spermatid to the mature spermatozoon is FSH-mediated. The maturation and acquisition of motility which occur in the epididymis are also androgen-dependent. Negative feedback of testosterone at the level of both the hypothalamus and pituitary control LH, and hence testosterone levels. Negative feedback by inhibin controls FSH levels. Thus, if there is destruction of the sertoli cells, and hence loss of inhibin, FSH levels will rise (Bain and Keene 1975).

Sperm transport in the male

The spermatozoa and the seminal plasma must be deposited in the vagina in close proximity to the cervix. Sperm transport occurs in two stages—that from the testes to the epididymis, and that from the epididymis to the vagina at the time of ejaculation.

Constant ciliary action and contraction in the wall of the seminiferous tubules move the spermatozoa and a small amount of tubular secretion through the tubuli recti to the rete testis, whence they pass to the epididymis. The spermatozoa remain within the epididymis for 20 to 30 days, during which time they undergo further maturation. Movement from the caput to the cauda of the epididymis is maintained by constant regular muscular contractions of the epididymal duct. At the time of ejaculation, mature spermatozoa are initially forced along the upper part of the vas deferens by contractions of this duct that are norepinephrine-mediated. Rhythmic contractions of the bulbocavernous and ischiocavernous muscles, which are innervated by the pudendal nerve, propel the semen along the urethra. At this time, the contributions of the prostate, the seminal vehicles, and the bulbourethral and urethral glands are added. The final mixing of the ejaculate occurs within the vagina and the cervical mucus (Jequier 1986).

While ejaculation can occur from a flaccid penis, erection is necessary for penetration and deposition of the ejaculate close to the cervix. Erection is mediated by vascular engorgement of the corpus spongiosum and corpora cavernosa of the penis. The vascular engorgement is mediated by the parasympathetic system.

THE INVESTIGATION OF SPERMATOGENESIS AND SPERM TRANSPORT IN THE MALE

For pregnancy to occur, spermatozoa in sufficient quantity must be produced, must transit the male ductal system, must negotiate the cervical mucus, uterine cavity, and fallopian tube, and, finally, must fuse with and fertilize the oocyte.

Those investigations aimed at defining the efficacy of the first two functions, production and transport in the male, will be described in detail in this chapter. The other aspects of sperm function mentioned will be discussed briefly here when relevant, and in greater detail in subsequent chapters.

The initial evaluation of male fertility is dependent upon

the history, the physical examination, and evaluation of the ejaculate.

History

This section will concentrate on those aspects of history-taking which have specific relevance to male fertility potential.

The age of the male partner should be noted, as fertility does decrease with age. Whether this is due directly to age, the age of the partner, or decreasing coital frequency is difficult to determine (James 1979). Whether or not the man claims previously to have fathered a pregnancy should be determined, and, if so, how long ago? The general state of health and social habits, including alcohol-, tobacco-, and other substance-abuse, are recorded. Any history of impotence or premature ejaculation is sought.

History-taking now moves to inquiries which may point towards specific causes for reduced male fertility. A logical series of questions progresses from prenatal influences to current events. Prenatally, exposure to diethylstilboestrol may cause both anatomical and spermatogenic abnormalities (Stillman 1982). Undescended testes as a child or post-pubertal mumps orchitis may be of poor prognostic significance (Lee and Lipshultz 1985). Delayed onset of puberty may hint at a chromosomal or endocrine abnormality. Inguinal herniorrhaphy, particularly in childhood, may have resulted in the inadvertent occlusion of the vas deferens. Testicular injury can depress spermatogenesis. A history of any sexually transmitted disease will raise suspicion for ductal occlusion, and is also relevant to the status of the partner's fallopian tubes. In adult life, particularly in the older patient, diabetic neuropathy, neurological disorders, and surgery of the bladder neck may lead to impotence and/or retrograde ejaculation (Seibel 1990).

Any severe endocrinopathy can depress spermatogenesis and is usually symptomatic. In particular, the sense of smell should be evaluated. If absent, Kallman's Syndrome (congenital hyposmia and hypogonadotrophinism) should be suspected. The need to shave daily, or the ability to grow a beard or moustache, is an excellent clinical indication that testosterone production is normal. Failure of sexual hair-growth indicates lack of androgen production in

Caucasian, Semitic, and Aryan patients. Such is not necessarily the case in those of African, Amerind, and Oriental origin.

As has previously been noted, during the 80 to 100 days taken by the sperm to mature a large number of systemic influences may be acting upon the spermatozoa. These include toxins, medications, radiation, exposure to excessive heat, and intercurrent infections (Seibel 1990).

Physical examination

If there is reason to suspect an endocrinopathy or a chromosomal abnormality, a thorough search for obvious physical stigmata should be sought. In particular, the sense of smell should be tested, and any gynaecomastia, decreased body hair, and eunuchoid proportions should be evaluated.

If the history is devoid of any obvious clues, an argument can be advanced for deferring physical examination of the male until after the initial semen analysis has been performed.

No useful information, other than that pertinent to routine health screening, was obtained in men with normal or subnormal seminal analysis (Dunphy *et al.* 1989*a*).

Such an approach clearly will prevent the discovery of varicoceles in a number of men with abnormalities of the semen analysis. Although early reports suggested a correlation between the finding of varicoceles and infertility (Dubin and Amelar 1971; Tulloch 1955), a well-performed study could find no difference in the incidence of varicocele in men with either normal or abnormal semen analyses (Nilsson *et al.* 1979). Nor must it be forgotten that the gold standard by which to measure the putative effect of any lesion upon fertility is whether or not pregnancy occurs. Rodriguez-Rigau *et al.* (1978) concluded that the presence or absence of a varicocele did not significantly alter the fertility outcome. Dunphy *et al.* (1989*a*) could show no correlation at the 5 per cent level of significance relating the chances of conception to whether or not a varicocele was detected. It is probable that a large number of men are submitted to unnecessary ligation of the spermatic vein (Baker *et al.* 1985). Until properly randomized studies comparing the occurrence of conception in women whose partners have been surgically treated with those whose partners have been managed conservatively are available, it is recommended that the search for, and the aggressive treatment of, varicocele is to be avoided.

In cases of ejaculatory dysfunction, suspected infection of the male accessory gland, or, if azoospermia has been detected, thorough examination of the male genitals should be performed. The evaluation of the genitals should note any anatomical abnormalities of the penis, including hypospadias and epispadias.

Testicular volume is estimated using an orchidometer (Prader 1966), and should be at least 20 ml. If the upper part of the epididymis is distended, obstruction is present. Hardness of the epididymis suggests that severe infection has occurred. The vas should be palpated. Congenital absence can occur. A rectal examination is usually only of value in patients with suspected obstructive azoospermia.

Evaluation of the ejaculate

From the perspective of the practising clinician, the whole purpose of evaluating the ejaculate is to determine the fertilizing potential of an individual male. Evaluation of the ejaculate, unless performed meticulously, is useless. Even the most accurate results from the most sophisticated laboratories, however, do not necessarily correlate with fertility.

This section will describe:

(i) the collection of the sample;

(ii) the performance of the classic semen analysis;

(iii) the interpretation of the results; and

(iv) the assessment of certain functional aspects of the spermatozoa.

Collection of the sample

The sample, produced by masturbation, should be collected into a sterile wide-mouthed container which is not spermatotoxic. Coitus interruptus will often loose the sperm-rich first portion of the ejaculate, and condoms are spermicidal. For those patients with religious or other constraints against masturbation, special silastic condoms are available. Specimens collected in such a way may show higher values than those produced by masturbation (Zavos 1985).

The period of sexual abstinence will influence the semen characteristics. The actual numbers will increase, but the motility will decrease with a longer time left between ejaculations. The sample should be collected after a three-day period of abstinence. The time of abstinence should be noted on the requisition form. All other clinically relevant data, including drug ingestion, recent illnesses, alcohol and tobacco intake, and other substance-abuse should also be recorded.

The classic seminal analysis

The fresh ejaculate is allowed to liquefy, and the time taken to liquefy is noted. Subsequent evaluation may be performed by classical microscopy or by the use of automated analysis systems. The measurements include volume, sperm density, motility, and morphology. After liquefaction has occurred, usually in about 20 to 30 minutes, the semen is pipetted and the volume is measured. A drop is placed on a microscope slide and covered with a coverslip. A phase objective lens and condenser are used for viewing at ×400.

If no sperm are seen in the sample, the whole specimen should be centrifuged at 2000G for ten minutes, and smears should be re-examined for the presence of sperm. If none are found, no further analysis can be performed, and the man is said to be 'azoospermic'. Aspermia describes a different condition, where no ejaculate is produced. Both conditions may indicate occlusion of the ductal system.

The wet slide is examined for spontaneous agglutination and clumping. The presence or absence of crystals, particulate debris, and cells other than spermotozoa is noted. (These other cells may be leukocytes, immature germinal cells, or epithelial cells.)

Sperm motility is assessed by examining five to ten microscope fields. The number of motile sperm per 100 sperm observed is counted twice, and the results are expressed as an average of the two values. The type of movement is also characterized, as (a) rapid, linear, and progressive; (b) slower and sluggish linear, or non-linear, movement; (c) non-progressive motility; and (d) immotile sperm (WHO 1987). The visual estimation of motility is usually inaccurate: the 95 per cent confidence interval for the estimated result is 30–60 percentage points (Amann 1979). If observers are meticulously trained, simultaneous assessments of motility by two observers can achieve a correlation coefficient of around 0.90 (Mortimer *et al.* 1986).

Next, an initial estimation of sperm density is made, and dilution of the sample should be carried out. The ratio of diluent to sperm is based upon values derived from these initial estimates of density (Mortimer 1985*a*). With some currently available observation chambers dilution of the sample is not necessary. The fine details of techniques for measuring sperm density can be found in the WHO laboratory manual (WHO 1987) or in an excellent review by Mortimer (1985*a*).

The morphology of the spermatozoa is assessed following fixing and staining (Mortimer 1985*a*). The shape and appearance of the human sperm cell have long been recognized to be variable among both fertile and infertile men, and human semen appears to contain a relatively high proportion of cells with abnormal appearance (Bostofte *et al.* 1985; MacLeod 1964; Sherins *et al.* 1977). Normal spermatozoa exhibit an oval-shaped head, with a regular outline and an acrosomal cap covering more than one-third of the head's surface. The head and mid-piece together are 10–13 μm in length, and the tail is at least 45 μm in length (WHO 1987). Morphological changes in the head are the most common abnormality of shape, and are more frequently associated than other deformations with clinical infertility (Bostofte *et al.* 1985; Sherins *et al.* 1977). Among the types of abnormality found in the head, tapered heads are most frequently observed; but round heads without an acrosome and other acrosomal anomalies account for a substantial proportion of the abnormal sperm.

The assessment of morphology is subjective, and variability between samples may range as high as 60 per cent (Zaini *et al.* 1985). Added to the expected biological variability, therefore, is a random error of measurement attributable to operator judgement; such judgement is called for more often because of the multiple categories of abnormalities that have been defined.

To try to overcome the inaccuracy inherent in the visual analysis of the sample, automated methods have been introduced. In addition to producing the same measurements as the classic analysis, these instruments will generate information about sperm movement characteristics. These movement characteristics will be discussed in detail in subsequent chapters.

Suffice it to say at this point that automated analysis holds promise of greater accuracy and reliability. To date, there are no data showing that sperm-density results obtained from the automated systems are superior to classic visual counting in the prediction of pregnancy. The automated equipment is expensive, and may only be available in centralized or research-based laboratories.

The interpretation of the results

In order to interpret the results published accurately, seminal analysis data must be correlated with fertility. As the gold standard of any test of fertility must be the occurrence or non-occurrence of pregnancy, the conclusions in this chapter will be derived from those studies based on infertile couples in which the test results were related to the subsequent occurrence of pregnancy. The finding of azoospermia clearly defines a given man as infertile. In the absence of such a finding, the clinician must make decisions based upon the best available information. The interpretation of the seminal analysis is fraught with pitfalls, not the least of which is the power of numbers. Physicians and patients alike are more comfortable with hard facts than with uncertainty. No facts are harder than numbers, the means by which semen-analysis results are expressed.

It is the purpose of this section to demonstrate that these apparently hard facts are some of the least accurate pieces of information available to the physician; yet in day-to-day practice we are still heavily dependent upon the results of the semen analysis in forming a clinical judgement. Better insight can be gained by pooling information from large numbers of reported studies. In order to pool this information it is necessary to submit the reported data to statistical analysis. A range of statistical methods may be of value in identifying the most useful clinical applications of the specific diagnostic tests. The section that follows will initially describe the principles of these statistical methods, and then these methods will be applied to the relevant studies that relate the diagnostic test to pregnancy outcome. The reader may find the detailed analysis of the raw data confusing; so the study results are presented in tables, and, it is hoped, in a clinically useful form. In preparing this material we abstracted the seminal and pregnancy data from the original publications, constructed two-by-two tables, and, finally, calculated the confidence intervals, test properties, and significance estimates.

When any diagnostic test is ordered, the physician should have two concerns (Feinstein 1977):

i. how well do the results of a specific test *predict* ubsequent outcome?

ii. how well do different tests *discriminate* between the desired outcome (in this case, fertility) and an alternative which is not desired (infertility)?

Generally speaking, diagnostic test properties based upon *prediction* are the most useful in clinical practice, and those that express *discrimination* serve as measures of quality, and are used to compare similar diagnostic tests one with another.

Diagnostic test are predictors for the presence or absence of disease, and so may be right or wrong; thus four results are possible:

(a) Abnormal test result, disease present = true positive;

(b) Abnormal test result, disease absent = false positive;

(c) Normal test result, disease present = false negative; and

(d) Normal test result, disease absent = true negative.

These results are usually arranged in the form of a two-by-two table (Table 4.1).

A perfect test would never have false positives or false negatives, and with unerring accuracy would predict the relevant outcome. Obviously no clinical tests achieve this level of accuracy. A series of terms have been introduced which describe how well a given test performs in the clinical setting (Table 4.2). As these measures of test performance will be applied throughout the text, each will be defined and its derivation described.

The terms positive predictive value and negative predictive value describe the ability of a test to forecast the outcome. No other test properties are more useful in clinical practice. Other test properties

Table 4.1 *Diagnostic test results and disease in the context of infertility*

	Disease present (infertility continues)	Disease absent (conception)
Test result abnormal	a (true positive)	b (false positive)
Test result normal	c (false negative)	d (true negative)

are needed, however, because predictive values may change in different clinical settings, as will be demonstrated. These other properties include sensitivity, specificity, and the likelihood ratios. As with the predictive values, a perfect test would have a sensitivity and a specificity of 100 per cent.

Although sensitivity and specificity are useful expressions of the quality of one diagnostic test compared with another, they are less useful to the clinician, because they work backwards from the diseased or non-diseased population to the test results.

The likelihood ratios allow us to compare the usefulness of abnormal results separately from normal results. The likelihood ratio of an abnormal test (LR+) expresses the greater probability that disease actually exists rather than does not exist if the text result is abnormal. Thus it is usually greater than one. Good test performance is associated with LR+ over 5; and an excellent test would be over 10 (Table 4.3).

The LR(−) expresses the likelihood of disease over non-disease when the test results are normal, and thus is usually less than one. Good tests would have an LR(−) of less than 0.5, and excellent tests one of less than 0.1. Clearly, the less the likelihood of disease with a negative test, the more accurate is the test (Table 4.3).

In the context of infertility, negative and positive predictive values, used in the strict sense, becoming confusing. A test with a good positive predictive value is accurate in identifying disease; at first sight it might be assumed that a good positive prediction

Table 4.2 *Diagnostic test definitions in the context of infertility*

Negative predictive value (NPV): the proportion of patients in whom a normal test result is found who are free of the condition.
Infertility context: the number with a normal test result who do conceive divided by the total with a normal result.
Formula: $d/c + d$.*

Positive predictive value (PPV): the proportion of patients in whom an abnormal test result is found who will actually suffer from the condition.
Infertility context: the number with an abnormal test result who do not conceive divided by the total with an abnormal test result.
Formula: $a/a + b$.

Sensitivity: the fraction of patients with the condition who have an abnormal test result.
Infertility context: the number with an abnormal test who do not conceive divided by the total not conceiving.
Formula: $a/a + c$.

Specificity: the fraction of patients who do not suffer from the condition who have a normal test result.
Infertility context: the number with normal tests who conceive divided by the total conceiving.
Formula: $d/b + d$.

Likelihood ratio of a positive (abnormal) test (LR+): the ratio of the likelihood of disease over the likelihood of non-disease, given an abnormal test.
Formula: sensitivity divided by (1 − specificity).

Likelihood ratio of a negative (normal) test (LR−): the ratio of the likelihood of disease over the likelihood of non-disease, given a normal test result.
Formula: (1 − sensitivity) divided by specificity.

---

* For definition of a, b, c, d, see Table 4.1

should relate to a good outcome, but such is not the case. The 'disease' here is the continuation of infertility. Thus a superior positive predictive value indicates a greater likelihood of a negative clinical outcome, or continuing infertility. Conversely, a superior negative predictive value predicts a better chance of the very positive outcome of pregnancy.

The clinician interested in infertility can easily sidestep this complexity. It is mathematically equivalent to express the predictive values in terms of pregnancy rates for normal and abnormal test results, which then can be compared.

Table 4.3 *The interpretation of likelihood ratios (LR+ and LR−) as expressions of the quality of a diagnostic test*

	LR+	LR−
poor	1.0 to 2.0	1.0 to 0.5
fair to good	2.0 to 5.0	0.5 to 0.2
good to excellent	5.0 to 10.0	0.2 to 0.1

These pregnancy rates are derived from clinical studies. In a study with large numbers, the estimated pregnancy rate is more likely to be accurate than is the rate derived from a small study. In order to account for this uncertainty, the 95 per cent confidence interval (CI) is calculated. The 95 per cent CI will be narrow in a larger study, and wider in a small study.

In order to compare pregnancy rates accurately, it is necessary to compare, not the observed rates, but the calculated 95 per cent CIs. If they overlap, the test results do not predict different outcomes.

While sensitivity and specificity are useful to compare one test with another, the clinician is more interested in predictive values. With the test result in hand, the clinician wishes to know the future probability of disease. After all, the advice given to the individual patient is based upon this information. Hence the pregnancy rates associated with abnormal and normal test results are of primary importance; but, as has been noted, these values may shift in different clinical settings, depending on the prevalence of disease, even though the sensitivity and specificity of the test remain constant.

The arithmetic in Table 4.4 illustrates how this shift can change the prediction of pregnancy when the test is applied to two different populations. This principle is important to the clinician who compares his or her experience with published reports. The reports will often be based on 'equal numbers' of diseased and non-diseased subjects; but the average clinical practice is rarely so judiciously distributed. Thus, whether disease prevalence is higher (as in the example) or lower in the practice, the published predictive values may not be confirmed by clinical experience.

It must be remembered that, just as predictive values can shift with prevalence, they can also shift according to the cutpoint at

Table 4.4 *How predictive values change with altered prevalence of disease, given that the sensitivity and specificity are constant and equal to 80 per cent*

	Population One	Population Two
Prevalence $(a + c)/200$	$100/200 = 50$ per cent	$160/200 = 80$ per cent
Sensitivity $(a/a + c)$	$80/100 = 80$ per cent	$128/160 = 80$ per cent
Specificity $(d/b + d)$	$80/100 = 80$ per cent	$32/40 = 80$ per cent
PPV	$80/100 = 80$ per cent	$128/136 = 94$ per cent
NPV	$80/100 = 80$ per cent	$32/64 = 50$ per cent

which a test is deemed to be normal or abnormal. Cutpoints which yield the best combination of sensitivity and specificity are the most useful in practice.

Another statistical test (the Kappa statistic, briefly discussed in Chapter 3) can be of value to express the overall agreement between a test result and pregnancy. Kappa expresses the extent of agreement beyond chance, and usually has a numerical value between zero and one. Kappa values of less than 0.4 represent poor agreement, 0.4 to 0.75, good agreement, and above 0.75, excellent agreement.

REPORTED DATA ON SEMINAL VARIABLES AND FERTILITY

The semen analysis is the bench-mark assessment of the male partner. The value of other investigations of the semen is dependent on the comparison of any new test with the semen analysis. How then should the results (seminal volume, sperm density, sperm motility, and sperm morphology) be interpreted?

One source of confusion is the wide variety of cutpoints used. Recommendations for the lower level of normal sperm density range from 5 to 60 million sperm per ml. Yet, when attempts are made to relate specific cutpoints to the occurrence of pregnancy, no clear correlations can be made (Collins 1989).

Nevertheless, to discard cutpoints entirely would result in chaos. A consensus statement has been made by the World Health Organization (WHO 1987), and it would seem reasonable to choose these values as arbitrary norms for use in clinical practice (Table 4.5).

Table 4.5 *Normal values of semen variables*

Ejaculate volume	2 ml or more
Sperm density	20 million per ml or more
Sperm motility	50 per cent or more with forward progression
Sperm morphology	50 per cent or more with normal morphology

Source: WHO 1987

How well these recommended norms perform in the clinical setting will now be discussed.

Volume (2 ml or more)

Reports of the correlation between seminal volume and pregnancy among infertile couples are infrequent. In one long-term study seminal volume was not correlated with time to pregnancy in the partners of men in either of two groups evaluated several years after seminal analysis (Bostofte *et al.* 1990).

Sperm density (20 million per ml or more)

Eight published studies have related sperm-density values to the occurrence of pregnancy. The number of couples in these studies ranged from 66 to over 1000, and totalled 3967; for one study, cumulative pregnancy rates have been used to construct two-by-two tables (Kjaergaard *et al.* 1990). Different cutpoints were used to define normal versus abnormal results. Table 4.6 summarizes the relationship between test results at given cutpoints and the pregnancy rates, with their 95 per cent confidence intervals. The frequency of an abnormal result, as defined by the author's cutpoint, is also shown in this Table. Not surprisingly, the lower the cutpoint the fewer the patients who were seen with abnormal results. Even in the larger series, there is overlap in the confidence intervals when the higher cutpoints (20 or 60 million) are used. Thus sperm-density results seem to allow some discrimination between those couples who will and those who will not conceive. However, the prediction is relatively inaccurate.

If a cutpoint at 5 million is used, the likelihood ratios are fair to

Table 4.6 *Sperm density as a predictor of pregnancy among infertile couples*

Cutpoint (10⁶/ml)	n	Pregnancy rates per cent (95 per cent CI)		Abnormal test frequency per cent	Authors
		Abnormal test	Normal test		
1	331	10 (0,21)	39 (33,45)	9	Johansson 1957
5	709	25 (13,37)	44 (40,48)	7	Peng *et al.* 1987
	783	23 (12,34)	58 (54,62)	7	Bostofte *et al.* 1982
	140	42 (14,70)	59 (50,68)	9	Smith *et al.* 1977
	1012	9 (6,12)	22 (19,25)	30	Stanwell-Smith and Hendry 1984
Weighted means (per cent)		**19**	**43**	**16**	
10	709	32 (22,42)	44 (40,48)	11	Peng *et al.* 1987
	1012	13 (10,16)	22 (18,26)	48	Stanwell-Smith and Hendry 1984
	705	42 (20,64)	73 (70,76)	3	Kjaergaard *et al.* 1990
Weighted means (per cent)		**27**	**48**	**21**	
20	709	34 (26,42)	45 (41,49)	18	Peng *et al.* 1987
	66	27 (1,53)	33 (21,45)	17	Shy *et al.* 1988
	783	41 (33,49)	59 (55,63)	17	Bostofte *et al.* 1982
	1012	17 (14,20)	19 (15,23)	66	Stanwell-Smith and Hendry 1984
	705	50 (40,60)	76 (73,79)	14	Kjaergaard *et al.* 1990
Weighted means (per cent)		**34**	**53**	**26**	
30	331	24 (17,31)	45 (38,52)	39	Johansson 1957
60	331	26 (20,32)	50 (42,58)	56	Johansson 1957
	709	38 (33,43)	47 (42,52)	48	Peng *et al.* 1987
	221	5 (0,10)	34 (26,42)	36	Macomber and Sanders 1929
Weighted means (per cent)		**30**	**45**	**47**	

good (2–5). When any higher cutpoint is used, the LR+ values are, with one exception (Macomber and Sanders 1929), less discriminating (Table 4.7). The negative likelihood ratios are poor (fair to good would be 0.2 to 0.5). The poor performance of a normal test is not surprising considering the almost limitless potential for some other cause of infertility, even among apparently normal infertile couples.

When the Kappa statistic was calculated (Table 4.7), it would seem that the agreement between sperm density and pregnancy is only marginally better than that which might be expected by chance (Kappa range 0.02–0.24, remembering that <0.40 represents poor agreement).

How can this information be used clinically? Obviously, the quality of the information does not allow a single-minded interpretation of any individual test result. The accumulated data suggest that the recommended cutpoint of 20 million sperm/ml is better applied to select men falling below this value who require further study than for the purpose of predicting pregnancy. A lower cutpoint, such as 5 million sperm/ml, can be used for the purposes of making a prediction, for men who fall below that value, that the chance of pregnancy is reduced. Even at this cutpoint, however, as the test quality is insufficient to permit an arbitrary decision, the results should be considered in the light of clinical information, such as the duration of infertility, and of other test results (Bostofte 1987; Dunphy *et al.* 1989*b*; Polansky and Lamb 1989; Small *et al.* 1987).

Motility (more than 50 per cent with progessive forward motility)

Table 4.8 illustrates the results of studies which compare motility with pregnancy. Patients reported by Bostofte *et al.* 1984 were followed by questionnaire for 20 years after assessment. They evaluated total motility of 20, 40, and 60 per cent cutpoints. All the other studies evaluated progressive motility. The confidence intervals of the pregnancy rates for normal and abnormal tests were only marginally separated, except in the study with the lowest cutpoint. In this study, however, only 3 per cent of men fell below the 20 per cent total motility level. Not surprisingly, the frequency of an

Table 4.7 *Diagnostic test quality: sperm density in the prediction of pregnancy among infertile couples*

Cutpoint (10^6/ml)	Likelihood ratios Abnormal test result	Normal test result	Kappa	Authors
1	5.4	0.89	0.08	Johansson 1957
5	2.2	0.94	0.05	Peng *et al.* 1987
	4.3	0.91	0.10	Bostofte *et al.* 1982
	1.9	0.94	0.06	Smith *et al.* 1977
	2.0	0.73	0.11	Stanwell-Smith and Hendry 1984
Weighted mean	**2.74**	**0.85**	**0.09**	
10	1.6	0.95	0.04	Peng *et al.* 1987
	1.4	0.76	0.09	Stanwell-Smith and Hendry 1984
	3.5	0.96	0.06	Kjaergaard *et al.* 1990
Weighted mean	**2.09**	**0.87**	**0.06**	
20	1.4	0.93	0.06	Peng *et al.* 1987
	1.2	0.96	0.02	Shy *et al.* 1988
	1.8	0.88	0.11	Bostofte *et al.* 1982
	1.0	0.92	0.02	Stanwell-Smith and Hendry 1984
	2.6	0.83	0.18	Kjaergaard *et al.* 1990
Weighted mean	**1.65**	**0.89**	**0.08**	
30	1.8	0.72	0.18	Johansson 1957
60	1.6	0.58	0.24	Johansson 1957
	1.2	0.85	0.09	Peng *et al.* 1987
	5.8	0.60	0.23	Macomber and Sanders, 1929
Weighted mean	**2.13**	**0.73**	**0.15**	

Table 4.8 *Sperm motility and pregnancy among infertile couples*

Cutpoint (percentage motile)	n	Pregnancy rates per cent (95 per cent CI)		Abnormal test frequency per cent	Authors
		Abnormal test	Normal test		
20	774	22 (6,38)	57 (53,61)	3	Bostofte et al. 1984*
25	709	36 (27,45)	49 (45,53)	15	Small et al. 1987
40	774	41 (31,51)	58 (54,62)	13	Bostofte et al. 1984*
50	709	39 (33,45)	52 (47,57)	40	Small et al. 1987
	286	42 (35,49)	41 (30,52)	72	Glazener et al. 1987c
Weighted means (per cent)	40	50	56		
60	66	26 (11,41)	29 (22,56)	53	Shy et al. 1988
60	774	50 (44,56)	60 (56,64)	40	Bostofte et al. 1984*
Weighted means (per cent)	47	58	47		

* Cutpoints at 20, 40, and 60 per cent for total motility among 774 men, followed by questionnaire 20 years after assessment; all other cutpoints refer to progressive motility.

Table 4.9 *Diagnostic test quality: sperm motility in the prediction of pregnancy among infertile couples*

Cutpoint* (percentage motile)	Likelihood ratios		Kappa	Authors
	Abnormal test result	Normal test result		
20	4.4	0.95	0.05	Bostofte *et al*. 1984*
25	1.5	0.93	0.06	Small *et al*. 1987
40	1.8	0.92	0.08	Bostofte *et al*. 1984*
50	1.4	0.82	0.12	Small *et al*. 1987
50	1.0	1.05	−0.01	Glazener *et al*. 1987*c*
Weighted means	**1.3**	**0.88**	**0.08**	
60	1.3	0.74	0.13	Shy *et al*. 1988
60	1.3	0.85	0.10	Bostofte *et al*. 1984*
Weighted means	**1.28**	**0.84**	**0.10**	

* Cutpoints at 20, 40, and 60 per cent for total motility among 774 men followed by questionnaire 20 years after assessment; all other cutpoints refer to progressive motility.

abnormal test increased as the cutpoint moved higher. Table 4.9 expresses the LR+, LR−, and Kappa values for these studies.

The likelihood ratio for an abnormal test (in the 3 per cent of men below the extreme cutpoint of 20 per cent) is satisfactory (4.4); but the Kappa value (0.05) indicates that the overall agreement between sperm motility and pregnancy is only 5 per cent better than chance alone. This is because the Kappa value also incorporates the experience of the other 97 per cent of individuals whose test results exceeded the cutpoint, in whom the test did not perform well (LR− = 0.95).

It could be suggested that the estimation of sperm motility would be more useful in some men than in others; where sperm concentrations are lower, the percentage with good motility could be more important. The relationship is not straightforward, however, as the type of sperm movement that is effective in cervical mucus may be less than optimal for the penetration of egg investments (Aitken *et al.* 1984). That may explain why two studies that made use of multiple regression survival analysis found no predictive value in conventional progressive motility assessment (Dunphy *et al.* 1989*b*; Polansky and Lamb 1989). In a subgroup of couples characterized by more than 48 months' duration of infertility and a normal female partner, it was grade II or sluggish motility that correlated with the pregnancy rate (Dunphy *et al.* 1989*b*). The assumption that rapid linear sperm motility is a superior form of sperm movement should be the subject of further study. With respect to the published data on motility, the predictive value of progressive motility is not as good as that of total motility; furthermore, only the lower cutpoints are useful for prediction of a reduced pregnancy rate. Values derived from higher cutpoints in sperm motility, as with higher cutpoints in sperm density, can only serve as crude indicators of the need for further investigation.

Morphology (more than 50 per cent of sperm have normal appearance)

Although a high percentage of abnormal sperm appears to be related to fewer pregnancies during follow-up (Bostofte *et al.* 1984; Glazener *et al.* 1987*c*), the relationship is not consistent (Shy *et al.* 1988; Zaini *et al.* 1985). Table 4.10 compares these four studies, with the data arranged according to cutpoint. For these data, it would appear that any cutpoint at 40 per cent of normal sperm or less would lead to test results with reasonable predictive value.

Table 4.11 shows an LR + of 8.0 and LR − of 0.95 if the cutpoint is set at 20 per cent of normal forms. Such low values occurred in only 3 per cent of men (Table 4.9). While a result below this cutpoint correlates well with the probability that no pregnancy will occur, the 97 per cent of values that are 'normal' above this cutpoint are useless as predictors.

Assessment of morphology is bedevilled by intra- and inter-patient variability and by observer error. Further, the number of morphologically abnormal sperm may not be relevant to normal fertilization, because the cervix acts as a functional filter for the removal of sperm with abnormal morphology (Gonzales and Jezequel 1985). Although round sperm cells lack acrosomes, other visible abnormalities of shape may simply be markers for movement disorders that could be more directly related to the decreased fertility (Morales *et al.* 1988). Abnormal sperm tend to swim more slowly than normal sperm, and either characteristic may decrease the ability to penetrate cervical mucus (Mortimer and Templeton 1982). The study of morphology in groups of men with specific abnormalities of sperm morphology may lead to more discriminatory tests.

Table 4.10 *Sperm morphology and pregnancy among infertile couples*

Cutpoint (percentage motile)	n	Pregnancy rates per cent (95 per cent CI) Abnormal test	Normal test	Abnormal test frequency per cent	Authors
20	781	14 (0,28)	57 (53,61)	3	Bostofte *et al.* 1985
40	781	34 (22,46)	58 (54,62)	8	Bostofte *et al.* 1985
50	134	51 (35,67)	49 (39,59)	29	Zaini *et al.* 1985
	709	51 (47,55)	39 (32,46)	70	Small *et al.* 1987
	286	41 (33,49)	64 (56,72)	51	Glazener *et al.* 1987c
Weighted means (per cent)		49	49	50	
60	781	48 (40,56)	58 (54,62)	21	Bostofte *et al.* 1985

Table 4.11 *Diagnostic test quality: sperm morphology in the prediction of pregnancy among infertile couples*

Cutpoint* (percentage normal)	Likelihood ratios Abnormal test result	Normal test result	Kappa	Authors
20	8.0	0.95	0.05	Bostofte *et al.* 1985
40	2.4	0.93	0.07	Bostofte *et al.* 1985
50	1.0	1.02	−0.01	Zaini *et al.* 1985
50	0.9	1.40	−0.10	Small *et al.* 1987
50	1.6	0.62	0.22	Glazener *et al.* 1987*c*
Weighted means	**1.05**	**1.16**	**−0.01**	
60	1.4	0.91	0.08	Bostofte *et al.* 1985

COMBINATION OF SEMINAL VARIABLES

From the foregoing, it is clear that single seminal variables considered in isolation are, at best, inaccurate predictors of a given man's fertility. In order to try to improve the predictive value, the combined effect of several variables can be studied. Such combined variables include:

  i. motile density (density/ml × percentage motile) (Glazener *et al.* 1987*c*; Hargreave and Elton 1986);

 ii. total motile sperm count (density/ml × volume × percentage motile) (Small *et al.* 1987; Smith *et al.* 1977);

iii. total normal motile sperm count (density/ml × volume × percentage motile × percentage normal forms) (Glazener *et al.* 1987*c*); and

 iv. total count (density/ml × volume) (Glazener *et al.* 1987*c*).

Table 4.12 shows the cutpoints for these variables, the pregnancy rates with normal or abnormal test results (with the 95 per cent confidence limits), and the abnormal test frequency. When the cutpoint of any of these variables is very low, thus identifying very few men as abnormal, there is a satisfying difference between the pregnancy rates with normal or abnormal test results. Table 4.13

Table 4.12 *Assessment of various combinations of seminal variables and occurrence of pregnancy among infertile couples*

Comment	Cutpoint $(10^6/ml)$	n	Pregnancy rates per cent (95 per cent CI) Abnormal test	Normal test	Abnormal test frequency per cent	Authors
motile density	0.1	279	7 (0,17)	37 (31,43)	10	Hargreave and Elton 1986
motile density	2	279	17 (8,26)	40 (33,47)	25	Hargreave and Elton 1986
motile normal density	4	286	30 (21,39)	57 (50,64)	38	Glazener *et al.* 1987*c*
motile density	5	286	26 (16,36)	55 (48,62)	24	Glazener *et al.* 1987*c*
total motile count	5*	709	25 (14,36)	45 (41,49)	9	Small *et al.* 1987
motile density	10	279	24 (17,31)	42 (34,50)	46	Hargreave and Elton 1986
total motile count	12.5*	140	23 (5,41)	64 (55,73)	16	Smith *et al.* 1977
total motile count	20*	709	30 (22,38)	46 (42,50)	19	Small *et al.* 1987
total count	25*	286	27 (11,43)	50 (44,56)	10	Glazener *et al.* 1987*c*

* Millions per ejaculate

Table 4.13 *Diagnostic test quality: various combination of sperm variables in the prediction of pregnancy among infertile couples*

Comment	Cutpoint (10^6/ml)	n	Likelihood ratios		Kappa	Authors
			Abnormal test result	Normal test result		
motile density	0.1	279	6.5	0.88	0.08	Hargreave and Elton 1986
motile density	2	279	2.5	0.78	0.15	Hargreave and Elton 1986
motile normal density	4	286	2.1	0.65	0.26	Glazener *et al.* 1987c
motile density	5	286	2.7	0.75	0.21	Glazener *et al.* 1987c
total motile count	5*	709	2.3	0.93	0.06	Small *et al.* 1987
motile density	10	279	1.6	0.71	0.17	Hargreave and Elton 1986
total motile count	12.5*	140	4.7	0.76	0.25	Smith *et al.* 1977
total motile count	20*	709	1.8	0.88	0.09	Small *et al.* 1987
total count	25	286	2.5	0.91	0.09	Glazener *et al.* 1987c

* Millions per ejaculate

demonstrates that with low cutpoints, the LR+ are in the fair to good range, but the LR−, as expected, are poor. Although these combinations of variables may summarize the seminal information into a neat package for purposes of discussion, they seem to add little to the predictive value of the single variables.

In yet another attempt to make sense of the semen analysis, three recent studies made use of multiple regression survival analysis. This technique evaluates the effect of several variables simultaneously, by entering the variables individually or in combinations (Bostofte *et al.* 1990; Dunphy *et al.* 1989*b*; Polanski and Lamb 1989). Among various methods for evaluating the influence of clinical factors on a dichotomous outcome such as pregnancy, proportional hazards analysis is superior, in that time to the event is taken into account (Cox 1972). Only one of these studies found a significant association between seminal variables (morphology and motility) and the prognosis (Bostofte *et al.* 1990). In the second of these studies, no relationship was found between seminal variables and the probability of conception, either in the unselected sample ($n = 1089$), or in a subgroup ($n = 210$) with no evident infertility disorder in the female partner (Polansky and Lamb 1989). In the third study, with the addition of other clinical variables such as duration of infertility in the subgroup analysis referred to earlier in the section on sperm motility, the only seminal variable which correlated with fertility was the number of sperm with sluggish motility. Surprisingly, this type of motility seemed to be related to a better prognosis (Dunphy *et al.* 1989).

Despite many years of observational studies, it is clear that the conventional criteria of sperm quality must be carefully interpreted for the purpose of predicting pregnancy among infertile couples. Indeed, Forsey and Hull (1989) have gone so far as to remark 'It is now clear that standard seminal analysis is of little clinical value except when "counts" are extremely low'.

CONCLUSIONS

Azoospermia affects approximately 5 per cent of male partners (Bostofte *et al.* 1982; Small *et al.* 1987). If either azoospermia or aspermia is detected, an explanation of infertility exists, and will require further investigation.

If sperm are present but in values below the lowest cutpoints (density is less than 5 million per ml, motility less than 20 per cent, and the number of normal forms is less than 20 per cent), little doubt can exist that, although spontaneous conception can occur, the probability of pregnancy is at least marginally lower; and it is reasonable to identify a male-factor contribution to the couple's infertility.

The greatest difficulties in interpretation arise when the values for some or all of the variables lie above the lowest cutpoint, but below the arbitrarily lower limits of normal set out for guidance in the World Health Organization manual (WHO 1987). While our understanding of the underlying mechanism and our ability to predict outcome in such circumstances are less than perfect, it would be inappropriate to include such couples in the category of un-explained infertility.

Refinements in testing procedures and a broader range of tests of sperm function when applied to such circumstances may ultimately allow better discrimination, so that, in future, some patients will move from this rather artificial category of 'male factor' into the unexplained group, and vice versa.

Definition

The second prerequisite to establishing the diagnosis of unexplained infertility is the demonstration of seminal analysis values that meet or exceed the following values:

- *Sperm density greater than 20 million per ml*
- *Progressive motility greater than 50 per cent*
- *Normal morphology greater than 50 per cent*

---

5 Physiology and investigation of sperm and oocyte transport in the female

Once ovulation has occurred and the spermatozoa have been deposited in the lower genital tract, the spermatozoa must travel to the ampulla of the fallopian tube. The oocyte and its surrounding cumulus must leave the follicle, enter the infundibulum of the tube, and be transported to the ampulla.

This section will examine the current understanding of the physiology and investigation of sperm and oocyte transport in the female.

PHYSIOLOGY

Sperm transport

The spermatozoa must enter and traverse the cervical mucus, uterine cavity, utero-tubal junction, isthmus, isthmic ampullary junction, and proximal ampulla of the fallopian tubes. This journey is in part a function of the female reproductive tract, and in part a function of the inherent motility of the spermatozoa.

After ejaculation, a coagulum forms, from which the sperm cells must escape. The majority do so after liquefaction has occurred, and some may be identified in the cervical mucus within 1.5 minutes of ejaculation (Mortimer 1985*b*). The spermatozoon uses its tail as a means of propulsion. The energy required for the tail to beat is provided by substrates (fructose, glucose, and mannose) which are acted upon by metabolic and glycolytic enzymes, situated in the tail, and respiratory enzymes, which are confined to the mitochondria (Moghissi 1984).

The uterine cervix, the thick muscular lower portion of the uterus, connects the uterine corpus to the vagina. The cervical canal, 2.5 to 3.0 cm in length and 7 mm in diameter at its widest point (Moghissi 1984), is bounded inferiorly by the external os and superiorly by the internal os. The endocervical canal is lined with columnar epithelium which possesses secretory capability, although there are no true glands. The epithelium is folded in an intricate pattern, the depressions of which are described as crypts (Fluhmann 1961).

The secretory epithelium of these crypts produces mucus at a rate of 20–60 mg/day, increasing to 700 mg/day at mid-cycle (Moghissi 1976*a*). Not only does the volume of mucus produced vary throughout the menstrual cycle, but so do certain physical attributes. The most important of these are *scinnbarkeit*, 'ferning', and cellular content. *Scinnbarkeit* describes the ability of fluids to be drawn into threads. 'Ferning' is the formation of crystals when the mucus is allowed to dry on a microscope slide (Papanicolaou 1946). Cells, predominantly leukocytes, appear within the cervical mucus. All of these phenomena are related to the cyclic production of oestrogen and progesterone. The degree of *scinnbarkeit* and ferning is low in the early follicular phase (low oestrogen), maximal in the immediately pre-ovulatory phase (high oestrogen), and virtually disappears in the luteal phase (oestrogen plus progesterone). The number of leukocytes which are detectable remains relatively high in the follicular phase, falls to its nadir on the day of the LH peak, and returns to a slightly higher than follicular level in the luteal phase. Other physical properties of cervical mucus, including viscosity, flow, elasticity, plasticity, and tack have been described. A full discussion is provided by Moghissi (1984).

Cervical mucus is a glycoprotein gel composed mainly of water (92 to 94 per cent), inorganic salts, low molecular weight organic compounds, high molecular weight compounds, enzymes, and proteins (Yudin *et al.* 1989). Penetration of this cervical mucus is the first step on the journey of the spermatozoon on its way to the ampulla. The ability of the sperm to penetrate the cervical mucus is a function both of the qualities of the mucus and the inherent motility of the spermatozoa. It is also possible that the cervical crypts may play a part as storage reservoirs for spermatozoa.

As the ejaculate comes in contact with the cervical mucus, the buffering capacity of the seminal plasma protects the spermatozoa from the highly acidic vaginal environment (Fox 1973). Penetration of the mucus by the spermatozoa begins almost immediately. The maximum number of spermatozoa is present in the cervix within 15 to 20 minutes of insemination (Tredway *et al*. 1978). This number remains constant for 24 hours, and declines thereafter; those spermatozoa which remain in the cervical mucus maintain their motility for 72 hours or more (Gibor *et al*. 1970; Gould *et al*. 1984).

Columns of spermatozoa, described as 'phalanges', form (Moghissi *et al*. 1964; Perloff and Steinberger 1963). It is possible that the differences in the pH of the vagina and the cervical mucus set up an electrical field which aligns the spermatozoa within the cervical mucus (Miller and Kurzrok 1932). The leading or vanguard spermatozoa seem to effect some changes in the cervical mucus which affect the motility of subsequent waves of invading sperm cells (Katz and Overstreet 1980). It has been postulated that the cervical mucus, as well as acting as a filter preventing the further progress of unhealthy sperm cells, also serves as a storage reservoir (Mattler 1973; Gould *et al*. 1984).

Channels form between the mucus macromolecules. It is probable that some of the spermatozoa, which must follow these channels, arrive in the crypts, which act as a cul-de-sac trapping the sperm cells. Only those sperm which enter channels leading to the internal os eventually proceed higher within the uterus and tubes (Mortimer 1983). Given receptive cervical mucus, transit of the cervical canal by spermatozoa is probably a function of their own propulsive efforts. This journey may be completed in about one to two hours following cervical deposition (Settlage *et al*. 1973).

Little is known about the mechanism whereby spermatozoa transit the uterine cavity. Uterine contractility may be involved, effectively mixing the sperm cells uniformly through the uterine fluid (Mortimer 1983). Recent observations have identified subendometrial myometrial contractility, moving towards the fundus in the immediately pre-ovulatory period (Lyons *et al*. 1991).

While information in the human is scanty, experiments in sheep and cows have provided information about tubal transport of spermatozoa (Hunter 1987). In sheep and cows, six to eight hours are required for spermatozoa to reach the fallopian tubes. They appear to be held in the very proximal isthmus (the interstitial portion in the human) for 17 to 18 hours, and are not released to travel to the site of fertilization until ovulation has occurred. Jansen (1978 and 1980) has identified a column of viscous mucus in this region of the tube in the pre-ovulatory period in the human. The concept of an isthmic reservoir (rather than a cervical one) is intriguing, given the need to delay some of the changes which the spermatozoa must undergo to effect fertilization. The only satisfactory human evidence for isthmic storage is the finding of spermatozoa in the distal ampulla 85 hours after coitus (Ahlgren 1975). At this time, the cervical complement of sperm cells is reduced (Gould *et al.* 1984).

The mechanism of passage of the spermatozoa from the isthmus to the ampulla is also unknown, but passage is probably effected by the combination of muscular and/or ciliary activity of the tube and the inherent motility of the spermatozoa (Mortimer 1983). Sperm cells enter the ampulla, and some ultimately will be found in the peritoneal cavity (Horne and Thibault 1962).

The numbers of spermatozoa at different levels of the genital tract decrease drastically from cervix to ampulla. This probably represents a process of natural selection, the less healthy cells falling by the wayside. It also ensures that excessive numbers are not present at the site of fertilization. Too many could result in polyspermic fertilization (Thibault 1972).

The time taken for spermatozoa to travel from cervix to proximal ampulla is probably of the order of 24 to 30 hours. Earlier results in animals suggesting a rapid transit phase of a few minutes only (Hafez 1973 and 1980) probably represent an experimental artefact, a subject discussed in greater depth by Mortimer (1983) and Hunter (1987).

Oocyte transport

The oocyte leaves the follicle surrounded by the cumulus mass. In the human there is no direct connection between the fallopian tube and the ovary. With respect to the events before fertilization, the tube is therefore responsible for oocyte pick-up, retention, and transport to the site of fertilization.

The tubes are paired muscular structures lying between the layers of the broad ligament. The distal extremities do not have a peritoneal covering. Anatomically, four regions are identified. The most distal portion, composed of frond-like fimbria, is the infundibulum. From the infundibulum, the ampulla gradually narrows until it joins with the isthmus. The isthmus terminates at the tubocornual junction, where the remainder of the tube, the interstitial portion, pierces the myometrium and opens into the uterine cavity. The muscular make-up and epithelial lining vary throughout the anatomical regions of the tube.

Oocyte pick-up is a function of the fimbria, although in experimental (Halbert and Patton 1981) and clinical situations (Novy 1980) oocyte pick-up can occur in their absence. At the time of ovulation, contractions of the fimbria ovarica and the infundibulopelvic ligament bring the fimbria into close approximation with the ovary. The oocyte and cumulus remain adherent to the follicles until they come into contact with the fimbria (Blandau 1969). Scanning electron microscopy has shown that the epithelial cells are richly provided with cilia (Halbert 1983). It is the action of these cilia upon the cumulus which propels the oocyte and cumulus mass towards the infundibular ostium.

Once in the ampulla, transport is relatively rapid. The actual time in the human is not known, but is probably in the region of the 30 minutes observed in monkeys (Blandau 1978). The mucosa of the ampulla, which is also richly ciliated, is lush and folded. There is little space between these folds. Despite earlier assumptions that ampullary retention and transport was a function of muscular peristalsis, it has been convincingly demonstrated that such is not the case (Blandau *et al.* 1979; Maia and Coutinho 1972). The large cumulus mass is in tight apposition with the cilia, and it is this ciliary action which seems to be responsible for transport. Once at the isthmic ampullary junction, the oocyte–cumulus complex will remain in the ampulla for about 72 hours (Croxatto *et al.* 1978). While the ampullary milieu is not essential to the occurrence of fertilization, which can be achieved *in vitro*, it probably provides the optimum environment. This ampullary retention is not due to a true anatomical sphincter, but rather to a combination of the passive mechanical properties of the ampullary and isthmic musculature, together with the difference in size between the oocyte–cumulus complex and the isthmic lumen, the actions of the cilia, and the effects of muscular contractions (Halbert 1983). For optimum oocyte pick-up and ampullary transport, therefore, there must be an unobstructed ovarian surface, freedom of the action of the infundibulum, patency of the infundibulum and ampulla, and a healthy ciliated endosalpinx.

INVESTIGATION

Sperm transport

The investigation of sperm transport in the female has largely concentrated on evaluation of the sperm–cervical mucus interaction, both *in vivo* and *in vitro*. Laparoscopic recovery of spermatozoa from the peritoneal fluid (Asch 1976; Ramsewak *et al.* 1990; Templeton and Mortimer 1980) has been proposed as a means by which the transit of the entire reproductive tract can be assessed.

The ability of sperm to penetrate cervical mucus is integral to the reproductive process, and reflects characteristics not only particular to the mucus but also to the spermatozoa. These interactions may be evaluated either *in vivo* (the post-coital test) or by a number of *in vitro* methods. Those *in vitro* methods using the partner's cervical mucus are testing both aspects of function. Those using mucus substitutes are testing sperm function only. Those which evaluate the quality of the mucus in isolation address only mucus characteristics.

History

There are few historical clues or physical findings, other than of a surgical procedure such as cone biopsy, which might have removed the cervical mucus-secreting epithelium, that suggest a potential causative factor for infertility attributable to poor-quality or absent cervical mucus.

The postcoital test

First described more than a century ago (Sims 1869), this test has become an integral part of the investigative protocol of many infertility practices. In simple terms, the cervical mucus is examined microscopically at a variable time following intercourse in the immediately pre-ovulatory period. The sample obtained is evaluated for the presence of spermatozoa. To be performed correctly, this preovulatory timing is of paramount importance, given the recognized variation in the properties of cervical mucus depending upon the hormonal environment. The standard unit of 'sperm per highpowered field' fails to take into consideration that the 'high-powered field' varies with different models of microscopes and with the type of eyepiece used. This fact alone makes comparison of published studies extremely difficult. The technique of performance of the *in vivo* postcoital test is described by Mortimer (1985*b*).

On the basis of their quantitative overview, Griffith and Grimes (1990) have concluded 'the post-coital test lacks validity as a test for infertility'. Hull *et al.* (1985) maintain that 'penetration of mucus is an essential test more discriminating than standard semen analysis provided that valid conditions are ensured'. Clearly, the value of this test is controversial. Given that in America the cost of one postcoital test is $50, it has been calculated that the annual cost in the United States for this single procedure is $50 million (Griffith and Grimes 1990).

The true value of any test for infertility is to predict whether or not pregnancy will occur. At first sight, there appears to be a positive correlation between the number of motile spermatozoa observed in the mucus and pregnancy (Collins *et al.* 1984; Harrison 1981; Hull *et al.* 1982*b*; Jette and Glass 1972; Samberg *et al.* 1985; Santomauro *et al.* 1972). The correlation is not strong, though, in results based on the most frequently used cutpoint, five sperm per high-power field (Fig. 5.1). The 95 per cent confidence intervals of the pregnancy rates with normal and abnormal test results frequently overlap. In four of six reports the Kappa statistic indicates that the agreement between postcoital tests and pregnancy is little better than would be expected from chance alone. In an evaluation of these and other reported studies Griffith and Grimes (1990) concluded that, although the predictive value of an abnormal test was superior to that of a normal test, neither was sufficiently accurate to indicate the appropriate clinical management.

Kovacs *et al.* (1978) reported that abnormal postcoital tests occurred

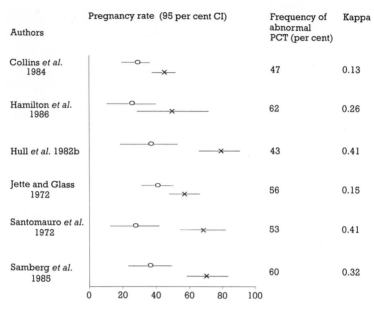

Fig. 5.1 *Correlation between postcoital test (PCT) results and pregnancy. Cutpoint 5 motile sperm per high-power field. Pregnancy rate (per cent and 95 per cent confidence interval (CI)): abnormal PCT: (—O—); normal PCT: (—×—).*

with equal frequency in women attending an infertility clinic and in women who recently had been delivered. Southam and Buxton (1956) found no sperm per high-powered field in 39 per cent of tests performed in conceptual cycles.

Regrettably, not only is the postcoital test a poor predictor of outcome, but abnormal results are observed with a very high frequency. In the previously cited papers, 43 to 62 per cent of the test results were abnormal. The agreement between the test and pregnancy outcome may be improved by repeated testing (Harrison 1981), but, even so, the results do little more than reflect the total motile sperm count (Collins *et al.* 1984). This information can be derived more easily from the semen analysis.

With regard to the purposes for which it was designed, 'to determine whether there is a sufficient number of active spermatozoa in the cervix but also to evaluate sperm survival and behaviour many hours after coitus (reservoir role)' (American Fertility Society 1986), the postcoital test leaves a certain amount to be desired.

In view of these data, and given the recognized psychological stress placed upon couples by this procedure (Harrison 1981; Drake and Grunert 1979), it is concluded that the *in vivo* postcoital test is stressful and provides little insight to assist one in defining a cause for infertility. This is not to say that disorders of cervical mucus do not cause infertility, but rather to emphasize that the *in vivo* postcoital test does not identify such disorders.

In vitro *tests*

The quality of the cervical mucus can be assessed by *in vitro* study of its physical properties. The sperm−mucus interaction can be studied by slide or tube tests using partner and/or donor mucus. Synthetic mucus substitutes can be used to evaluate the ability of spermatozoa to penetrate.

Physical properties

Assessment of the oestrogenic effect on cervical mucus can be carried out by naked eye and microscopic examination. A scoring system has been developed (Insler *et al.* 1972). Numerical values are assigned to the degree of dilatation and the condition of the external os, the amount of mucus, *scinnbarkeit*, ferning, and the number of leukocytes present. (This last criterion was added after the original scoring system was developed.) A maximum score of 15 is attainable. A score of 12 or more indicates good pre-ovulatory cervical mucus. Complete details of the performance of this test are described by Mortimer (1985*b*).

When evaluated clinically, it has been found that cervical mucus characteristics are excellent in most women when timed accurately, and do not correlate with the occurrence of pregnancy (Collins *et al.* 1984; Pandya *et al.* 1986; Schats *et al.* 1984).

Sperm−mucus interaction

Placing a drop of semen in contact with a drop of cervical mucus on a microscope slide (Kurzrok and Miller 1928) is the oldest *in vitro* method of assessing sperm—mucus interaction. The degree of penetration of the spermatozoa is assessed, and is expressed as 'normal' or 'abnormal'.

Sperm and mucus can be mixed and observed (Sperm—Cervical-Mucus Contact (SCMC) Test) (Kremer 1965). If the sperm are seen to exhibit 'shaking' phenomenon, there is a high correlation with the presence of anti-sperm antibody. This subject will be addressed in Chapter 8.

The capillary tube test (Kremer Test) is performed using the female's mucus in a flat capillary tube, the open end of which is placed in a reservoir of the male partner's semen. After one hour, the depth and degree of sperm penetration is recorded (Kremer 1968). An empirically derived semi-quantitative score is assigned from 0 to 16. Scores are interpreted as 0 = negative, 1 to 9 = poor, 9 to 11 = average, 12 to 15 = good, ⩾ 16 = excellent.

The crossed hostility test (Kremer 1968; Moghissi 1984) is usually only performed if the score on the Kremer test is less than 12. This test consists of paired Kremer tests, where two columns of the patient's mucus are inserted into preparations of partner and donor semen and two of donor mucus are similarly placed. In theory, at least, such a test should discriminate between failure of penetration due to mucus causes and that due to spermatic causes. Difficulties in obtaining donor mucus render the test impractical.

Mucus substitutes, including bovine cervical mucus (Alexander 1981), polyethylene glycol bisacrylate (Bissett 1980) and polyacrylamide gel (PAG) (Lorton *et al.* 1981) have been investigated to assess sperm—mucus-substitute penetration ability. Results in human cervical mucus and surrogate media, such as bovine mucus and polyacrylamide gel, have indicated that these media may have value as substitutes for human mucus (Bissett 1980; Collins 1987; Goldstein *et al.* 1982; Mortimer 1985*b*; Overstreet 1986). Human sperm tend to penetrate further in human cervical mucus (mean = 55 mm) than in bovine mucus (mean = 23 mm), and the prognostic value of human mucus penetration is superior to that of bovine mucus penetration (Eggert-Kruse *et al.* 1989*b*). An evaluation of polyacrylamide gel (PAG) revealed that, while the estimate of sperm penetration distance was precise, this information was not useful in the prediction of pregnancy (Gwatkin *et al.* 1990).

Although mucus penetration results correlate with sperm motility and other estimators of fertility, the prediction of pregnancy among groups of infertile couples based on the use of bovine and synthetic gels is not associated with discriminating test results (Collins 1989*a*). It must be stressed that sperm—mucus or sperm—mucus-surrogate penetration tests give little information about the cervical mucus, but are another means of assessing spermatic movement. Although the movement of sperm through cervical mucus is essential for fertilization, the optimal test for evaluating this sperm function remains undecided. Studies are necessary to demonstrate the relative value in clinical practice of the various methods available for estimating sperm movement, which include progressive motility, swimming speed, lateral head deviation, and mucus penetration. It is becoming increasingly important to know to what extent the various measurements reflect identical or distinct movement characteristics.

Assessment of sperm transport from the uterus to the ampulla

Attempts have been made to recover spermatozoa from uterine washings (Maathuis and Aitken 1978). It is extremely difficult to obtain specimens which are free from mucoid contamination (Mortimer and Templeton 1982). Such techniques are not yet applicable in clinical practice.

In 1962, Horne and Thibault described the recovery of spermatozoa in peritoneal fluid washings. The ability to recover such spermatozoa gives some indication of the functional integrity of the sperm-transport mechanism in women with patent fallopian tubes. Interestingly, although clearly no sperm can enter tubes which are occluded at the tubo-cornual junction, large numbers can be found in the fluid contained in hydrosalpinges (Ahlgren 1975).

Laparoscopy performed in the immediately pre-ovulatory period can be used to attempt such sperm recovery (Asch 1976; Ramsewak *et al.* 1990; Templeton and Mortimer 1980, 1982). Positive sperm recovery had a good correlation with pregnancy (Mortimer and Templeton 1982), and negative sperm recovery held a poor prognosis. Ramsewak *et al.* (1990) studied 15 couples with evidence of normal ovulation, seminal analysis, and bilateral tubal patency.

Spermatozoa were recovered laparoscopically in all 15 women. Given the logistical difficulties in scheduling the operating room at short notice to perform laparoscopy at the appropriate time to attempt laparoscopic sperm recovery, and the relative paucity of data, this test of sperm transport must await further validation.

Oocyte pick-up and ampullary transport

Most major insults to the fallopian tubes follow either infective or traumatic events. Traumatic events may include intra-abdominal surgical procedures and intrauterine manipulations (Taylor and Graham 1982). As the investigations of individual couples will progress at differing speeds, clinical indication of urgency in investigation of tubal structure would be valuable. The investigations available primarily assess tubal patency and gross tubal architecture. Early attempts to use radioactive microspheres (Pauerstein *et al*. 1977) as oocyte surrogates to evaluate oocyte transport were not clinically valuable. Recently, Uher *et al*. (1990) have introduced biodegradable microspheres into the pouch of Douglas either by laparoscopy or by cul-de-sac puncture. These were collected in a cervical cap 24 hours later. The microspheres, which were recognizable by fluorescence, were demonstrable in the cap in 66 per cent of 69 patients with unexplained infertility, and in 100 per cent of 20 patients with male-factor infertility. This report suggests a further avenue of investigation. Fimbrial microbiopsy has proved insufficiently representative of the total picture of the tubal mucosa to be of prognostic significance (Brosens and Vasquez 1976).

The investigative procedures presently available include hysterosalpingography and laparoscopy, of which, at present, laparoscopy is the reference procedure (Collins 1988). How well do laparoscopic findings correlate with clues detected in either the history or physical examination?

Table 5.1 demonstrates the correlation between historical or physical findings and the presence or absence of an intrapelvic abnormality. Although these clinical factors have some predictive value, it must not be forgotten that up to 75 per cent of patients with hydrosalpinges will exhibit neither a history of pelvic pain or pelvic infection nor positive physical findings (Rosenfeld *et al*.

Table 5.1 *Clinical factors as predictors of pathological findings during laparoscopy among infertile couples*

Clinical factor	Percentage with abnormal findings at laparoscopy (95 per cent CI)		Kappa value
	Factor absent	Factor present	
Pelvic pain	37 (25,49)	81 (64,98)	0.32†
Appendectomy	37 (25,49)	59 (40,78)	0.19†
D&C	37 (25,49)	65 (44,86)	0.10†
History positive*	32 (27,37)	69 (61,77)	0.33†
Abnormal pelvic examination	40 (35,45)	80 (68,92)	0.15‡
Duration of infertility more than six years	40 (35,45)	57 (46,68)	0.11‡

* History positive for any of: pelvic infection, intrauterine device, endometriosis, ovarian surgery, or tubal surgery.
References: † Cumming and Taylor 1979; ‡ Portuondo *et al*. 1984.

1983). The history and physical examination are indirect evidence only, and a negative history and negative physical findings do not preclude the presence of intrapelvic lesions. As fallopian tube obstruction, much of which is asymptomatic, will occur in 12 to 33 per cent of infertile couples (Collins *et al*. 1983; Hull *et al*. 1985; Kliger 1984), early investigation of tubal patency is indicated. With respect to unexplained infertility, while a demonstration of tubal occlusion clearly demonstrates a probable cause of infertility, tubal patency does not ensure functional integrity.

Fallopius described the structures as 'tubae' (Latin 'trumpets') resembling as they did the straight trumpets of classical Rome. Modern transliteration of 'tubes' has led to the perception of a long, narrow, hollow structure, requiring patency only to function. Translation of 'trumpet', with its complex array of curves and valves, would better have expressed the complexity of tubal function.

Hysterosalpingography (HSG) is a simple, non-operative, radiological procedure which may demonstrate lesions of the uterine cavity and fallopian tube. (Lesions of the uterine cavity will be discussed in Chapter 10. This section will be confined to discussing the investigation of the tubes.)

In principle, the technique simply involves the instillation of a radio-opaque fluid into the uterine cavity and, using image intensification, the observation of the passage of this fluid through the cavity and along the fallopian tubes. Early and delayed X-ray films are exposed. A detailed description of technique is provided by Hunt and Siegler (1990). The procedure is not entirely risk- or pain-free (Marshak *et al.* 1950). Pain can be reduced by prior administration of a prostaglandin synthetase inhibitor. Marked bradycardia may develop (SanFillippo *et al.* 1978). The most significant risk is the reactivation of quiescent pelvic inflammatory disease. This may occur in approximately 3 per cent of patients (Stumpf and March 1980). This is a serious event, given that the risk of sterility rises from 13 per cent after one episode of tubal infection to 36 per cent after two (Westrom 1975). To combat this risk some centres prophylactically administer antibiotics. Factors which would identify women at risk include a history of prior infection or surgery, adnexal tenderness or enlargement, and those in whom secondary infertility has been identified. These factors would have predicted reinfection in 50 per cent of the women who suffered this event (Stumpf and March 1980). Although the consequences of reinfection are serious, the 3 per cent incidence is sufficiently low to suggest that routine treatment prophylaxis is not necessary for all women. Women in the high-risk group or in whom cervical cultures are positive for the recognized pathogens might be treated with antibiotics; but, given the greater likelihood of pelvic lesions being present, laparoscopy may be a preferable test in such patients.

The radio-opaque material for HSG may be oil- or water-soluble. While water-based media demonstrate the tubal mucosal patterns more effectively (Alper *et al.* 1986), there may be a higher pregnancy rate in women with unexplained infertility when an oil-based medium is used (DeCherney *et al.* 1980; Schwabe *et al.* 1983). The question of whether these conceptions represent the passage of the contrast medium or simply the passage of time remains to be answered.

Laparoscopy and dye transit are performed under general anaesthesia. The technique is described in detail by Steptoe (1967) and Gomel and Taylor (1986). The procedure is not without risk. A mortality rate of 11 per 100 000 diagnostic laparoscopies was reported in 1974–5 (Phillips *et al.* 1976). A complete description of the complications will be found in Gomel *et al.* (1986).

The lesions detected by this technique are shown in Table 5.2. Periadnexal adhesive disease, usually not identified by hysterosalpingography, can be observed through the laparoscope. These periadnexal adhesions, if occurring in the presence of patent tubes, are not an absolute cause of sterility. Adhesions may reduce the likelihood of pregnancy, and may constitute an explanation of infertility. Whether they interfere with oocyte pick-up by encasing the ovary or restricting tubal movement, or are simply a visible indicator of more subtle damage to the function of the tube, is unclear. It is probable that both mechanisms are contributory.

Given that laparoscopy is the gold standard by which the final assessment of tubal status is made, it has been argued that immediate recourse to laparoscopy should supersede hysterosalpingography (Templeton and Kerr 1977; Taylor and Cumming 1979). Table 5.3 compares the laparoscopic with the hysterosalpingographic findings in several reported series.

In these series, the Kappa statistic indicated substantial agreement between the two procedures, even though HSG was not a perfect predictor of tubal occlusion as determined by laparoscopy. Further, these studies represent a selected population of patients in whom the aggregate prevalence of tubal occlusion was 38 per cent. This prevalence figure falls to 10 per cent in studies of large numbers of unselected patients (Collins *et al.* 1983; Hull *et al.* 1985), which more accurately represents the general population.

If in the average practice the prevalence of tubal obstruction is approximately 10 per cent, then the predictive value of the HSG may differ from the reported estimates in Table 5.3. The weighted means for sensitivity and specificity in the published data were 76 and 83 per cent respectively, and these test properties do not change from shifts in prevalence. The weighted means can be applied to a hypothetical group of 100 patients, in which 10 per cent have tubal obstruction, to give the results shown in Table 5.4. The calculations indicate that, in the average practice, a normal HSG will be followed by an abnormal laparoscopy in only 3 per cent of cases, and thus provides about 97 per cent confidence that an immediate laparoscopy is not required. A normal test result would occur in the majority (77 per cent) of patients. In the remaining 23 per cent of patients, an abnormal test result would require follow-up by lapar-

Table 5.2 *Infertility-associated pathology observed during laparoscopy procedures among infertile female partners*

Number of subjects	Abnormal findings (per cent)					Authors
	Tubal defect	Endometriosis	Leiomyomata	Other defects	Total defects	
675	27	8	4	2	41	Duignan et al. 1972
168	43	5	0	10	57	El-Minawi et al. 1978
215	46	5	5	10	65	Ismajovich et al. 1986
171	46	8	1	1	56	Kliger 1984
197	39	6	2	8	54	Liston et al. 1972
433	45	16	0	9	70	Nordenskjold and Ahlgren 1983
168	51	1	1	3	57	Philipsen and Hansen 1981
497	43	21	0	0	64	Taylor 1985
279	30	5	1	3	39	Templeton and Kerr 1977
Weighted mean	38	11	2	4	54	

Table 5.3 *Tubal obstruction as observed at laparoscopy: frequency associated with normal and abnormal HSG*

Number in study; and percentage with obstruction (bracketed figure)	Laparoscopic evidence of fallopian tube obstruction (per cent) and 95 per cent CI		Kappa value	Authors
	Normal HSG	Abnormal HSG		
Water-soluble contrast medium				
111 (29)	10 (7)	58 (15)	0.50	Gabos 1976
215 (25)	13 (6)	47 (11)	0.37	Ismajovich *et al.* 1986
50 (54)	24 (17)	84 (14)	0.60	Keirse and Vandervellen 1973
132 (48)	18 (9)	78 (10)	0.61	Moghissi and Sim 1975
326 (23)	8 (4)	46 (9)	0.41	Nordenskjold and Ahlgren 1983
152 (36)	10 (6)	77 (11)	0.68	Philipsen and Hansen 1981
336 (29)	10 (4)	70 (9)	0.61	Portuondo *et al.* 1980
143 (49)	16 (8)	84 (9)	0.68	Rice *et al.* 1986
143 (19)	11 (6)	44 (17)	0.36	Swolin and Rosencrantz 1972
121 (60)	32 (14)	73 (10)	0.38	WHO 1986
Weighted means				
1729 (33)	12 (2)	65 (4)	**0.54**	

Table 5.3 (*contnd.*)

Number in study; and percentage with obstruction (bracketed figure)	Laparoscopic evidence of fallopian tube obstruction (per cent) and 95 per cent CI		Kappa value	Authors
	Normal HSG	Abnormal HSG		
Medium oil-soluble or not stated				
273 (25)	6 (3)	72 (10)	0.69	Duiggan et al. 1972
352 (30)	10 (4)	76 (8)	0.66	El-Minawi et al. 1978
108 (69)	58 (12)	84 (11)	0.24	Goldenberg and Magendantz 1976
409 (20)	6 (3)	65 (9)	0.62	Hutchins 1977
79 (58)	45 (22)	63 (12)	0.15	Idris and Jewelewicz 1976
84 (61)	16 (13)	88 (9)	0.72	Ladipo 1976
207 (38)	17 (7)	72 (1)	0.55	Maathuis et al. 1972
121 (15)	3 (3)	63 (19)	0.66	Servy and Tzingounis 1978
Weighted means				
1633 (32)	12 (2)	73 (4)	0.61	

Weighted mean: sensitivity of HSG = 76 per cent; specificity of HSG = 83 per cent.

Table 5.4 *Predictive value of HSG in an infertility practice with prevalence of tubal obstruction equal to 10 per cent*

| | Laparoscopy results | | Total |
	Obstructed	Patent	
HSG results:			
Abnormal (obstruction)	7.6[a]	15.3[b]	23[a+b]
Normal (patent)	2.4[c]	74.7[d]	77[c+d]
Total	10.0	90.0	100

Calculations: [a] = 76 per cent (sensitivity) × 10; [c] = 10 − 7.6;
[d] = 83 per cent (specificity × 90; [d] = 90 − 74.7
pPV = 7.6/23 = 33 per cent, (67 per cent of abnormal HSG results
will be proved wrong at laparoscopy);
NPV = 74.7/77 = 97 per cent, (97 per cent of normal HSG results
will be proved right at laparoscopy).

oscopy, at which time the result would be more likely than not to be proved wrong, as the laparoscopic findings would be normal. Aggregate data thus allow a smooth transfer of diagnostic information to the practice setting, where the prevalence of disorders such as tubal obstruction and endometriosis may be quite different from the prevalence in published reports.

The data support a rational approach to the investigation of tubal patency, using the HSG as a screening test for low-risk couples. If the X-ray is abnormal, laparoscopy should be performed. Those in whom the hysterosalpingogram is normal may wish to defer laparoscopy for six months in the hope that spontaneous pregnancy will occur. Those at high risk, with a history of pelvic infection and abnormal pelvic findings, or with prolonged infertility, or with the age of the female partner greater than 35 years, should forgo HSG and immediately undergo laparoscopy.

Intra-tubal polyps may be identified by hysterosalpingography. David *et al.* (1981) have suggested that they might cause infertility. Prospective studies by Glazener *et al.* (1987*d*) have shown that the likelihood of conception is no different in women with otherwise unexplained infertility whether tubo-cornual polyps are present or not; nor has surgical excision of these lesions improved the chances of pregnancy (Gordts *et al.* 1983).

CONCLUSION

Failure of sperm or oocyte transport within the female tract would cause infertility. Unfortunately, the *in vivo* postcoital test lacks validity as a test for sperm transport in cervical mucus. Also, the application of *in vitro* sperm–cervical-mucus testing, even though the test may suggest the presence of anti-sperm antibody, is presently of dubious clinical value. Further research of typical patient populations may clarify the value of such *in vitro* mucus tests. Laparoscopic sperm recovery is not a practical clinical test.

Proximal tubal occlusion will inhibit sperm transport, and distal occlusion or periadnexal tubal disease will inhibit oocyte pick-up. Tubo-cornual polyps are not a cause of infertility. Except in defined cases, the preliminary evaluation of tubal patency should be by hysterosalpingography. In selected cases, and in those with abnormal hysterosalpingograms, laparoscopy should be performed immediately. In low-risk cases in whom the hysterosalpingogram is normal, laparoscopy should be deferred for six months in the hope that spontaneous pregnancy will occur. Nevertheless, infertility with respect to oocyte transport cannot be defined as unexplained until a laparoscopy has been performed.

Definition

Because of the present limitations of the tests which could evaluate sperm and oocyte transport in the female, the only valid observation is as follows: if the fallopian tubes are patent and free from adhesions, an impediment to sperm and oocyte transport has not been demonstrated. If such is the case, then with respect to sperm and oocyte transport, the infertility is unexplained. This diagnosis can only be made with confidence once a laparoscopy has been performed.

6 Fertilization and early embryonic development

INTRODUCTION

Crucial to the successful initiation of pregnancy are fertilization, early embryonic development, transport to the uterine cavity, and further embryonic development therein. This chapter will focus upon the physiology of these events and the clinical investigations which may be used to gain insight into these phenomena. Identifiable recurrent defects in any of these processes would provide an explanation for the couple's infertility.

DEVELOPMENT OF THE OOCYTE

It is worth remembering that the human oocyte, recovered from the fallopian tube washings, was not described until 1928 (Allen *et al*. 1928). Most of the information with respect to the early development of the human oocyte and embryo is derived from *in vitro* studies of oocytes produced as a result of hyperstimulation with either clomiphene citrate and/or human menopausal gonadotrophins.

The oocyte, immediately before the onset of the LH surge, lies within the follicle. It is surrounded by a mass of cells, the cumulus mass, the inner layer of which constitutes the corona radiata. Cellular processes from the cumulus can be seen penetrating the outer membrane of the oocyte. This close association between the oocyte and the cumulus is critical to oocyte maturation. Oocytes cultured in the complete absence of cumulus cells have almost no developmental capacity (Crosby *et al*. 1982). The cumulus cells play a major role in protein synthesis (Osborn and Moor 1982). Beneath the outer membrane of the oocyte, the zona pellucida, lies the perivitelline space. The oocyte plasma membrane separates the ooplasm from the perivitelline space.

Prior to the LH surge, the oocyte has not completed the first meiotic division. At the time of the LH rise, the final stages of the first meiotic division begin. The germinal vesicle breaks down, the first polar body containing the excess chromatin forms, and the oocyte chromosomes become rearranged on the second metaphase spindle. The cells of the cumulus mass assume a translucent appearance and become more loosely displaced. Concurrent with, but independent from the completion of meiosis, metabolic changes take place within the oocyte, the most obvious of which are the beginning of migration of the cortical granules to the periphery (Zamboni 1970) and an increase in the number of mitochondria (Masui and Clarke 1979). These metabolic changes are stimulated by the action of the gonadotrophins, which must act through the cumulus cells, as the oocyte lacks receptors for LH and FSH (Crosby and Moor 1984).

Immediately before follicular rupture the junctions between the cumulus and the oocyte break down (Gilula *et al.* 1978). The first polar body has been extruded, and the second meiotic division has reached metaphase. Attempts to fertilize an oocyte at this stage of development are usually unsuccessful *in vitro* (Edwards *et al.* 1969). A further three to six hours are required in the *in vitro* situation before maturation is completed.

The final maturation that renders the oocyte fertilizable is a complex mechanism. At least four interdependent events contribute to this process: the engulfment of the sperm head, the exocytosis of cortical granules, disintegration of the sperm nuclear envelope, and the condensation of sperm chromatin (Bedford 1981).

FURTHER DEVELOPMENT OF THE SPERMATOZOA

Freshly ejaculated spermatozoa are not capable of effecting fertilization. Attempts to perform *in vitro* fertilization of rabbit oocytes were unsuccessful until the spermatozoa had been exposed for some time to the secretions of the genital tract of the doe (Chang 1951; Austin 1951). This change in the spermatozoa is described as capacitation.

Capacitation appears to effect subtle changes in the spermatozoal membranes. Substances in the seminal plasma and possibly the cervical mucus inhibit capacitation, probably by binding to the membranes of the spermatozoa. The secretions of the female genital tract, particularly of the fallopian tube of the human, may be responsible for removing these inhibitors (Austin 1975). Given that the viability of spermatozoa rapidly decreases after capacitation has occurred, this is an elegant mechanism by which longevity is preserved until the spermatozoa are in close apposition to the oocyte. Direct identification of capacitated spermatozoa is difficult, although, clearly, if fertilization or oocyte membrane binding can be observed, it can be inferred that capacitation has occurred.

Light microscopy will not reveal the membrane changes, but changes in lectin binding and fluorochrome labelling have been described (Singer *et al.* 1985; Cross and Overstreet 1987). The most obvious change occurs in the motility patterns. The sperm become 'hyperactivated' (Yanagimachi 1988). The sperm head is observed to thrash rapidly from side to side, with no forward progression of the cell. Once capacitation has occurred the spermatozoa can now undergo the acrosome reaction. The acrosome is that region of the sperm head which is bound by the acrosomal membrane. The outer acrosomal membrane lies immediately below the plasma membrane, and the inner is adjacent to the nuclear membrane. The inner and outer acrosomal membranes fuse at the equatorial segment or acrosomal collar.

The acrosome reaction involves fusion of the inner and outer membranes at localized points, formation of membranous vesicles, and the release of enzymes stored within the acrosome (Edwards 1980). The two most important enzymes are hyaluronidase and acrosin. The acrosome reaction occurs when the spermatozoon is in close contact with the oocyte. Occurrence prior to penetration of the cumulus may be detrimental (Yanagimachi 1988).

The acrosome reaction can be detected by transmission electron microscopy, lectin, monoclonal or polyclonal antibody labelling (Mortimer *et al.* 1989; Yanagimachi 1988), or by inference if zona binding or penetration can be observed.

FERTILIZATION

At the time of fertilization, probably less than 500 capacitated spermatozoa surround the oocyte–cumulus complex (Mortimer 1983). The spermatozoa must penetrate the cumulus and the zona pellucida to enter the perivitelline space. Concurrently, the oocytes must prevent further spermatozoa from entering, otherwise polyspermic fertilization will occur. Penetration of the cumulus is in part effected by the hyperactive motility of the sperm head and in part by release of proteolytic enzymes. The zona is probably softened by the action of acrosin. Final penetration is effected by a mechanical cutting action of the sperm head. This cutting action is driven by the hyperactivated flagellar beating (Mortimer *et al.* 1989).

Once in the perivitelline space, the sperm head is bound to the vitelline membrane at the equatorial segment of the acrosome. It is the binding which triggers the activation of the oocyte, a phenomenon which is marked by the release of the cortical granules. The contents of these granules prevent further sperm penetration of the zona and block polyspermic fertilization (Sathananthan and Trounson 1982; Shabanowitz and O'Rand 1988).

The sperm head, having been taken into the ooplasm by a phagocytic mechanism, then decondenses and forms the male pronucleus. Simultaneously, a membrane forms around the female chromosomes, creating the female pro-nucleus. The two pro-nuclei fuse (syngamy), and the male and female chromosomes come together on the metaphase spindle of the first cleavage division. *In vitro*, the pro-nuclei can be identified about 12 to 18 hours, and fusion of the pro-nuclei 20 to 24 hours, after insemination (Trounson *et al.* 1982). At this point, fertilization is said to have occurred (Mohr and Trounson 1984).

EARLY EMBRYONIC DEVELOPMENT

Once syngamy has occurred, the zygote begins a rapid process of mitotic cellular division referred to as cleavage. The zygote will have become a two-cell embryo about 20 to 30 hours after insemination *in vitro* (Mohr *et al.* 1983). Subsequent cleavage will produce 4-, 8-16-, and 32-cell embryos, at which point the embryo is described as a 'morula'. A fluid-filled cavity begins to form, and cell division continues. The embryo containing the fluid-filled cavity is now the blastocyst. This stage of development is observed 90 to 100 hours after insemination *in vitro* (Edwards 1980).

The ultrastructural changes occurring between syngamy and blastocyst formation have been described in detail (Sathananthan 1984), but fundamentally involve regular cleavage with a reduction in cell size, nuclear activation, mitochondrial development, and development of intercellular communication. Differentiation of the cells into those which will form the embryonic and those which will form the trophoblastic tissues occurs (Mohr and Trounson 1984).

The human blastocyst hatches from the surrounding zona pellucida 140 to 160 hours after insemination (Edwards 1980). At the time of hatching, trophectoderm, primitive endoderm, and the inner cell mass can be identified (Mohr and Trounson 1984).

These changes may occur *in vivo* both in the fallopian tube and in the uterine cavity. The oocyte (and presumably, if fertilization has occurred, the zygote and early embryo) reside in the ampulla for 72 hours following ovulation. Transit through the isthmus is rapid, and takes only eight hours. Thus tubal transit time from ovulation to arrival in the uterine cavity is about 80 hours (Croxatto and Ortiz 1975). The mechanism of isthmic transport is unknown, but may involve alterations in the properties of the isthmic mucus (Jansen 1980). Relaxation of the isthmic musculature and reappearance of isthmic cilia are progesterone-mediated (Leeton and Kerin 1984). The roles of the components of the tubal fluid in sustaining the embryo are unclear; but it is likely that these are not critical, or successful pregnancy after *in vitro* embryonic maturation would not occur.

IMPLANTATION

On the basis of information derived from 15 human embryos recovered from uterine washing before implantation had occurred, Croxatto *et al.* (1979) demonstrated that the embryo had developed to the stage of a 12- to 16-cell morula on arrival in the uterine cavity. As it continues to develop to the blastocyst stage the embryo lies freely in the uterine cavity for a further three days. Thus about 6 days (132 to 144 hours) will have elapsed between fertilization and implantation (Hearn *et al*. 1988).

The embryo is active during this interval and begins to send signals of its presence to enable the maternal system to recognize the pregnancy. Human chorionic gonadotrophin (HCG) is identifiable as early as seven to eight days after fertilization (Hearn *et al*. 1988). A number of early pregnancy factors (EPF), including platelet inhibiting factor (PIF), can be identified at about this time (Morton *et al*. 1980).

Concurrent with the transport and development of the embryo, changes are occurring in the maternal endocrinological system and within the endometrium. In the non-conceptual cycle, corpus luteal function begins to decline eight to ten days after the mid-cycle LH surge. This is reflected in falling peripheral levels of oestrogen and progesterone. In a conceptual cycle, there is sustained luteal secretion of oestrogen, progesterone, and 17 α hydroxy progesterone. These changes are probably mediated by HCG secreted by the embryo. Adequate steroid secretion by the corpus luteum is necessary for implantation and sustenance of the early pregnancy for the first seven to nine weeks, after which time placental hormone production takes over these functions (Csapo *et al*. 1972). HCG levels, detectable from about 8 days after the LH surge, double every 2.5 days (Lenton *et al*. 1982).

The morphological and metabolic changes in the human endometrium in a conceptual cycle are, for obvious reasons, poorly understood. Changes occur in the concentrations of oestrogen and progesterone receptors, prolactin, and prostaglandins. The composition of the uterine fluid, in which the early blastocyst is bathed, also alters. This subject is reviewed in depth by Findlay (1984).

CLINICAL IMPLICATIONS

The processes of fertilization, early embryonic development, transport to and development within the uterus, maternal recognition of pregnancy, and implantation are complex. Not surprisingly, these processes may go awry.

Fecundability, the percentage of women exposed to the risk of pregnancy for one menstrual cycle who will produce a live-born infant, is only 15 to 28 (Short 1979). While these figures are discouraging for infertile couples, it must not be forgotten that there are presently in excess of four billion people on this over-crowded planet. Teleologically, this low rate of fecundability makes a great deal of sense.

Low human fecundability may in part be accounted for by failure of fertilization to occur, but also reflects a high rate of early-pregnancy wastage. Estimates suggest that 70 per cent of all conceptions fail to survive. Fifty-five per cent are lost before it is clinically recognized that pregnancy has occurred, and 15 per cent are clinically diagnosed as miscarriages (Findlay 1984). It is probable that, in normal women, very early pregnancy loss contributes more to the low fecundability rate than does failure of fertilization.

Clearly, a recurrent failure of any of the processes involved in fertilization and early embryonic development would constitute an explanation for infertility. How then are these processes investigated?

INVESTIGATIONS

Assuming that no obvious defects have been identified in male or female gametogenesis and gamete transport, there is little to be detected in the history or physical examination that might indicate defects of fertilization or early embryonic development. (A history of recurrent spontaneous pregnancy-loss might imply such defects; but habitual abortion is beyond the scope of this monograph.) Investigation of these processes is dependent upon the accessibility of the function to be studied. Although spermatozoa are readily available, fertilization and subsequent events can only be evaluated by *in vitro* fertilization (IVF). While IVF may provide insight into the fate of a given oocyte, the composition of a specific aliquot of follicular fluid, or a particular cohort of embryos, such observations are not reproducible or clinically practical as routine investigations. Similarly, maternal recognition of, and preparation for pregnancy, cannot be evaluated on a day-to-day basis.

This section will examine those clinical investigations, primarily of the spermatozoa, which relate to fertilization. The present state of knowledge with respect to the oocyte, its environment, and early embryonic development will be discussed briefly.

Spermatic function

The shortcomings of the classic seminal analysis and sperm–cervical-mucus interaction testing have been described. In order better to understand spermatic function, particularly with respect to its ability to effect fertilization, investigations of some aspects of function have been developed, which include:

  (i) sperm movement characteristics;

 (ii) biochemical properties;

(iii) interactions with cervical mucus;

(iv) assessment of capacitation and the acrosome reaction;

 (v) oocyte penetration and zona binding assays; and

(vi) *in vitro* fertilization.

Sperm movement characteristics

The automated systems for semen analysis described in Chapter 4 can also determine a number of movement characteristics. Those currently believed to be important are:

1. *Velocity*: the time taken to travel between two points.

2. *Linearity*. Sperm swim in a sinuous fashion. Linearity is calculated by measuring the length of the sinuous track of a sperm cell as it travels between two points. The straight-line distance between the two points is divided by the distance actually travelled. Clearly, a cell which has a limited amount of sinuous movement will have travelled less distance than one with exaggerated movements. Its path will be more 'linear'.

3. *Lateral head displacement*. As the sperm swims, the head moves from side to side. Measurement of the distance moved laterally by the sperm head from the straight-line path of sperm movement is described as 'lateral head displacement'.

At present, evaluation of these characteristics remains in the developmental phase, because the correlation between sperm movement characteristics and pregnancy is not strong enough to serve a diagnostic purpose. Among 68 couples with unexplained infertility, when sperm movement characteristics were evaluated, the mean velocity among those conceiving (24.6 ± 1.1 μm/second, $n = 24$) was similar to that observed among couples continuing without conception (23.6 ± 1.1 μm/second, $n = 38$) (Aitken *et al.* 1984). The concentration of spermatozoa with an amplitude of lateral head displacement less than 10 μm was also similar in the fertile and infertile groups. A recent report suggests that automated estimates provide no additional advantages over conventional semen analysis for the purpose of predicting pregnancy (Check *et al.* 1989). The continuing study of sperm movement may in the future strengthen the diagnostic evaluation of the infertile male.

Biochemical properties

The biochemical assessment of seminal fluid may serve to investigate:

  (i) the accessory glands;

 (ii) sperm integrity; and

(iii) certain functional aspects of the spermatozoa.

The accessory glands

Acid phosphatase, citric acid, zinc, and magnesium are specifically secreted by the prostate, fructose and prostaglandins by the seminal vesicles, and L-carnitine, glyceryl-phosphorylcholine, and 1-4 glucosidase by the epididymis (Jequier 1986). With the exception of L-carnitine and fructose, the estimation of which may be of value in cases of azoospermia, none of these substances is clinically informative about spermatic function.

Sperm integrity

Glutamic-oxaloacetic transaminase (GOT) and an isoenzyme of lactic dehydrogenase (LHD-C4) are released into the seminal plasma when spermatozoa die. Their clinical usefulness has yet to be established (Jequier 1986).

Functional aspects

The concentration of L-carnitine may be related to motility (Bornman *et al.* 1989). Clinical capacity of the assay is yet to be determined. Fructose is a necessary substrate for the anaerobic metabolism of spermatozoa. Absence of fructose will result in severely decreased motility, and is indicative of congenital absence of the seminal vesicles.

The biochemical estimation of adenosine triphosphate (ATP) may be more closely related to formulating a prognosis for infertile couples. The energy required for sperm-tail movement is generated from a complex intracellular economy through the breakdown of ATP. The concentration of ATP in the ejaculate is correlated with sperm density, although the expected correlation with sperm motility is not always present (Calamera *et al.* 1982; Comhaire *et al.* 1983; Irvine and Aitken 1985; Levin *et al.* 1981). In comparative studies, ATP concentration was significantly lower in the semen of infertile men compared with matched fertile donors (Comhaire *et al.* 1983). ATP estimates corrected for turbidity were marginally lower in fertile ejaculates compared with infertile ejaculates (Irvine and Aitken 1985).

The concentration of ATP in semen has been evaluated further with respect to follow-up in three studies, one of which found that the ATP concentration was correlated with sperm count, motility, and morphology; but this variable was not selected as a predictor of pregnancy during follow-up in a multivariate discriminant analysis (Wang *et al.* 1988). In the other studies, the role of prognostic factors was evaluated by survival analysis, and no statistically significant relationship at the 5 per cent level was observed in any group or subgroup between ATP concentration and conception (Dunphy *et al.* 1989*b*; Gwatkin *et al.* 1990).

Given the complexity of the sperm cell, compounded by the heterogeneity of sperm cells within a single ejaculate, it is not surprising that a single component of a major enzyme system has not revealed a clear and consistent correlation with pregnancy during follow-up. Because motility is an essential sperm function that is highly dependent upon energy supply, biochemical investigations which reflect this sperm function would have promising clinical applications. For example, sperm creatine phosphate kinase activity measured in raw specimens and after sperm migration appears to reflect the relative concentrations of a normal sperm subpopulation (Huszar *et al*. 1988). The search for a simple but discriminating variable that will express a critical aspect of sperm motility function and lead to a more accurate prediction of fertility is a high priority for andrological research.

Interaction with cervical mucus

The technique and correlation in both *in vitro* and *in vivo* sperm–mucus interaction tests have been described in Chapter 5. These tests are poor predictors for pregnancy.

Assessment of capacitation and the acrosome reaction

These functions can be assessed directly or by inference. The observation of hyperactive motility is indicative that capacitation has occurred, and zona binding or penetration is evidence that the acrosome reaction has taken place. Direct methods (lectin and chlorneotetracycline labelling) of identifying capacitation have yet to be evaluated sufficiently to permit assessment of their clinical value (Mortimer *et al*. 1989). Assessment of the acrosome reaction by transmission electron microscopy or various staining techniques must be carried out using dead cells. This being so, it is difficult to determine whether or not the acrosome reaction which is detected represents a genuine physiological event or simply post-mortem changes (Mortimer *et al*. 1989). It is therefore by direct observation that the fertilizing ability of spermatozoa is assessed.

Oocyte penetration and zona-binding assays

Sperm penetration assay (SPA)

The successful penetration by human sperm of the denuded hamster oocyte is a test of the ability of sperm to undergo the acrosome reaction and fuse with plasma membranes (Aitken 1983; Yanagi-machi 1984). In outline, the test is performed by super-ovulating golden hamsters with pregnant mare serum (Yanagimachi *et al.* 1976). The oviducts are removed and the oocytes expressed. The cumulus mass is dispersed with hyaluronidase and zonae digested with trypsin. Zona binding is species-specific, so the ability of the spermatozoa to penetrate heterologous oocytes can only be tested once the zonae have been removed. After incubation with prepared, and presumably capacitated acrosome-reacted spermatozoa, the oocytes are squashed under a coverslip and examined microscopically for the presence of swollen sperm heads within the ooplasm.

The prognostic value of the sperm penetration essay in the evaluation of male infertility and in the selection of patients for *in vitro* fertilization has been disappointing (Collins 1987; Mao and Grimes 1988). Numerous variations of the basic methodology exist, as would be expected during the development of a bioassay that requires the meticulous preparation of both male and female gametes. The variability in results may, to a certain extent, reflect these different test conditions.

In earlier reports, SPA results appeared to be correlated with pregnancy rates during follow-up among infertile couples. With no known female factors, abnormal SPA test results were associated with lower pregnancy rates (10 to 20 per cent) than were observed among couples with normal test results (42 to 47 per cent) (Aitken *et al.* 1984; Sutherland *et al.* 1985). When the test results are expressed as the number of sperm per oocyte, however, there is no consistent correlation with fertility (Gwatkin *et al.* 1990; Hargreave *et al.* 1988). Table 6.1 summarizes the published data, in which the test results are expressed as the percentage of hamster oocytes penetrated. The 95 per cent confidence intervals for the pregnancy rates associated with abnormal and normal results overlap or touch in every case, regardless of the cutpoint. The Kappa values indicate that agreement between the test result and fertility is poor, and yet the likelihood of an abnormal test result, which would require some explanation for the couple, is approximately 40 per cent (Table 6.2). Thus the sperm penetration assay as it is currently performed has little clinical value. When the results are expressed as a penetration index, one report revealed higher pregnancy rates associated with

Table 6.1 *Human sperm penetration in hamster oocytes as a predictor of pregnancy among infertile couples*

Cutpoint*	n	Pregnancy rates per cent (95 per cent CI)		Authors
		Abnormal test	Normal test	
1	149	7 (1,13)	19 (10,28)	Sutherland *et al.* 1985
10	66	19 (6,32)	48 (30,66)	Shy *et al.* 1988
	68	20 (4,36)	47 (32,62)	Aitken *et al.* 1984
	227	18 (10,26)	34 (26,42)	Corson *et al.* 1988
	227	15 (7,23)	19 (13,25)	Gwatkin *et al.* 1990
20	227	13 (7,19)	23 (15,31)	Gwatkin *et al.* 1990
25	68	29 (15,43)	48 (29,67)	Aitken *et al.* 1984

* Percentage of hamster oocytes penetrated

Table 6.2 *Tests of quality for human sperm hamster oocyte penetration assay in prediction of pregnancy among infertile couples*

Cutpoint*	n	Kappa	Frequency of abnormal results (per cent)	Authors
1	149	0.10	46	Sutherland *et al.* 1985
10	66	0.30	56	Shy *et al.* 1988
	68	0.23	37	Aitken *et al.* 1984
	227	0.14	44	Corson *et al.* 1988
	227	0.03	31	Gwatkin *et al.*1990
20	227	0.09	47	Gwatkin *et al.* 1990
25	68	0.19	60	Aitken *et al.* 1984

* Percentage of hamster oocytes penetrated

abnormal test results than with normal test results (Hargreave *et al.* 1988). None of the likelihood ratios are better than fair (Table 6.2).

Zona-binding assay

The ability to bind to zona of oocytes of the same species should reveal a great deal about the functional capacity of the spermatozoa (Yanagimachi *et al.* 1979). This bioassay has certain shortcomings:

the supply of human zonae required for this test is limited, and aging alone is sufficient to stimulate the release of cortical granules by human oocytes, which will effectively block zona-binding. This test awaits validation in the human.

In vitro fertilization

The ultimate test of spermatic function, and indeed of oocyte function, is the ability to effect human fertilization *in vitro*. If fertilization fails to occur, it can only be due to defects in the sperm, the oocyte, or the culture technique. Inseminating half the oocytes with partner's sperm and half with donor sperm in the same culture system should in theory address such questions (Wood *et al.* 1984). Such observations, however, can only allow tentative conclusions to be drawn from one particular test, and do not necessarily reflect sperm or oocyte quality in subsequent cycles. From a pragmatic point of view, it would seem reasonable, once a couple has gone so far as to attempt *in vitro* fertilization, to draw some clinical conclusions. If fertilization of healthy-appearing oocytes fails to occur when other tests of sperm quality and function have been suspect, the infertility might be attributed to the male factor. In couples in whom the male is apparently normal, and where fertilization has failed to occur, no such conclusions can be drawn. If the use of donor semen is acceptable to the couple, half the oocytes in a subsequent treatment attempt can be inseminated by donor insemination. This may identify a previously unsuspected male factor if the partner's sperm fails to fertilize but donor sperm is successful. But in this situation it is not unusual for all oocytes to be fertilized during the second attempt, and thus the cause of the infertility is no clearer.

The oocyte and its environment and early embryonic development

Since the introduction of the widespread use of *in vitro* fertilization (Steptoe and Edwards 1978) a great deal has been learned about oocyte quality and early embryonic development *in vitro*. Oocyte quality is assessed morphologically, mature oocytes being regular in shape, pale-coloured, and surrounded by 'activated' cumulus cells

(Mohr and Trounson 1984). The normal and abnormal development of embryos *in vitro* are beyond the scope of this review, but are described in great detail by Mohr (1984) and Edwards (1980). While these techniques have added greatly to our understanding of the complexities of the process of fertilization and early development in the human, they are of little help in further refining the diagnosis of unexplained infertility.

CONCLUSIONS

Given the low fecundability of the human and the complexity of fertilization, it would be surprising if recurrent defects in these processes were not causative of infertility. At present, few conclusions can be drawn when trying to establish an explanation for an individual couple's infertility. None of the clinical tests described in this chapter is sufficiently well developed to be useful in establishing a diagnosis of unexplained fertility.

Definition

Failure of spermatozoa, which previously have been judged abnormal by semen analysis or other tests of sperm function, to effect fertilization in vitro *can, for practical purposes, be said to explain a couple's infertility. Failure of apparently normal spermatozoa to do so if donor spermatozoa are effective may likewise implicate the male.*

While defects of fertilization and early embryonic development must be causative in some cases, the means of accurately detecting such defects have yet to be described.

---

7 Endometriosis

INTRODUCTION

Endometriosis could be a cause of infertility or it could arise as a result of prolonged failure to conceive. It is also possible that an underlying defect causes both endometriosis and infertility through independent mechanisms. Whether infertility in the presence of endometriosis can be unexplained is the subject of this chapter. The lesion was first described by Rokitansky in 1860, and even today no unified theory can account for the development of the condition (Ridley 1968). Stated simply, endometriosis is the finding of endometrial tissue (glands and stroma) in sites other than the uterine cavity. Even this simple definition is less than accurate. Morphological studies have demonstrated similarities between the ectopic and the normally situated tissues (Roddick et al. 1960). Significant differences are noted when specimens are examined by electron microscopy (Schweppe and Wynn 1981) and in the ability of the receptors of the endometriotic tissue to accept oestrogen and progesterone (Gould et al. 1983; Vierikko et al. 1985).

The lesions are extremely variable when observed with the naked eye. They range from a single spot within an otherwise apparently healthy pelvis to total pelvic disorganization caused by dense adhesion-formation and intra-ovarian cysts. Even when apparently healthy pelvic peritoneum is excised and examined microscopically, the typical histological pattern has been identified in 6 per cent of women complaining of infertility (Nisolle et al. 1990).

The most comprehensive system of classification (American Fertility Society 1985) recognizes four stages, from minimal to severe. Numerical values are assigned to the findings within these groups. The numerical score is from 1 to 114, attesting to the protean nature of the lesions. It is widely accepted that endometriosis of sufficient severity to cause pelvic disorganization, and hence probably to interfere with oocyte pick-up, is a cause of infertility. Thus, if such Stage III and IV lesions are identified, an explanation for the infertility exists.

The situation is much less clear with respect to State I (minimal) and Stage II (mild) endometriosis. Many questions remain unanswered. It has long been recognized that endometriosis is more prevalent in women who have not borne children. This immediately poses the question, does minimal or mild endometriosis cause infertility, or does childlessness simply permit the lesions to develop? This chapter will address this question by examining the aetiology of endometriosis and the potential mechanisms whereby its presence might interfere with fertility. A further method of answering the question 'Does a condition cause infertility?' is to asssess the effects of randomized trials of treatment versus no treatment upon subsequent pregnancy. These trials will be discussed. The methods of investigation necessary to establish a diagnosis of endometriosis will be described. The definition of unexplained infertility with respect to the presence or absence of endometriosis will be developed.

AETIOLOGY

Schweppe (1988) remarks that 'The histogenesis is poorly understood; the etiology unknown.' The major theories of causation for the presence of visible disease are implantation of endometrial fragments, which reach the pelvic cavity by retrograde menstruation (Sampson 1927), and metaplasia of the coelomic cells (Meyer 1919). In addition, haematogenous and lymphatic spread are possible (Sampson 1925).

It is probable that both major mechanisms contribute; but why, when retrograde menstruation has been demonstrated to occur in 90 per cent of 52 women with patent tubes (Halme *et al.* 1984*a*), do some but not all develop endometriosis? Genetic factors may play some role. A familial relationship has been demonstrated (Simpson *et al.* 1980). Immunological differences have been identified in some women with endometriosis. T-cell mediated cytotoxicity to endometrial tissue was reduced in patients with endometriosis when compared to age-matched endometriosis-free infertile controls (Steele *et al.* 1984). In women with the disease, complement levels are higher in both serum and peritoneal fluid, and macrophages are more numerous in peritoneal and tubal fluids (Badawy *et al.* 1984*a*; Haney *et al.* 1983; Muscato *et al.* 1982).

Dmowski *et al.* (1988) have suggested that the development of endometriosis may be due to a defect in the immune system. They postulated that the ability to deal with endometrial fragments shed during retrograde menstruation is a function of the peritoneal macrophages. If this system is overwhelmed or deficient, implantation of endometrial fragments might occur. The production of auto-antibodies to the endometrial cells could follow.

Some of the histological lesions may be influenced by the ovarian sex steroids. The ability of the cells to respond to endogenous oestrogen and progesterone varies widely, and is related to the ability of the cells to develop receptors (Schweppe 1988). Thus a mechanism can be postulated which implies that, in women with ineffective macrophages, lesions will develop, and the subsequent growth and dissemination of the lesions will then be dependent upon their ability to metabolize sex steroids. While this is a tidy hypothesis, there are large gaps in our understanding, and it fails to take into consideration the recognized possibility of coelomic metaplasia.

The histological appearances of the lesions, their distribution within the pelvis, and the association of endometriosis with other lesions of the genital tract, such as fibroids and congenital malformations, are well recognized, and will not be described here. The interested reader is referred to Schmidt (1985), Schweppe (1988), and Ramzy (1983).

PREVALENCE

Neither the incidence (annual occurrence) nor the prevalence (proportion of the populated affected) of endometriosis is known. The minimal standards of diagnosis require the observation of lesions at the time of either laparoscopy or laparotomy (Yuzpe *et al.* 1986), and the gold standard is the histological evaluation of tissue samples. Until a simple screening test is developed, the true incidence and prevalence of minimal disease in the total population will remain unknown.

Present information, therefore, is based upon prevalence studies in selected subjects. Collected data have shown ranges of 1 to 50 per cent in gynaecological laparotomies, 5 to 53 per cent in laparoscopies, and 15 to 24 per cent in women complaining of otherwise unexplained infertility (Schweppe 1988). Retrospective studies of asymptomatic women undergoing laparoscopy for sterilization suggest that endometriosis affects two to four per cent of such patients (Schweppe 1988). It is unlikely that such studies reflect the true prevalence of the condition in the general population. In the first place, the great majority of such subjects are parous, and pregnancy has a recognizably curative effect on endometriosis. The thoroughness with which a laparoscopic total pelvic survey was performed in these studies is unclear. Verkauf (1983) evaluated this question in a prospective study in which gynaecologists were specifically instructed to look for endometriosis at the time of laparoscopy in infertile women and in those undergoing sterilization. The prevalence in the infertile group was 39 per cent, and in the sterilization group it was 5 per cent. Nevertheless, until the incidence and prevalence of the disease in the total population are known, it will be imprudent to rely on selective prevalence figures to justify any conclusion that minimal or mild endometriosis can cause infertility.

A non-causal association with infertility is equally plausible. Mahmood and Templeton (1991) observed endometriosis during 21 per cent of 654 laparoscopies for infertility, compared with 6 per cent of 598 laparoscopies for sterilization. In these women and 290 others having laparoscopies for abdominal pain (156) or hysterectomies for bleeding (134) there was a higher frequency of endometriosis after a long interval either before or after child-bearing. Thus, among susceptible women, both fertile and infertile, endometriosis may develop as a result of prolonged exposure to uninterrupted menstruation.

POTENTIAL MECHANISMS OF CAUSATION OF INFERTILITY

Moderate and severe disease can interfere with fertility by purely mechanical means. For example, adhesions surrounding the ovaries or the tubes may inhibit tubal oocyte pick-up. No such simple explanation exists in lesser states of endometriosis, if the tubes are patent and the tubes and ovaries are free of adhesions. A number of alternative potential mechanisms have been described, and include:

(a) alterations in the peritoneal fluid;

(b) immunological disorders; and

(c) hormonal disturbances.

Alterations in peritoneal fluid

Various constituents of the peritoneal fluid, such as prostaglandins, might affect tubal function, fertilization, early embryonic development, or the endocrine function of the ovary.

Prostaglandin levels are difficult to measure, as the compounds have a very short half life. The volume of peritoneal fluid varies throughout the cycle, peaking in the immediately pre-ovulatory period (Maathuis *et al.* 1978). These two sources of variability may have confounded the results of prostaglandin studies. The differences in peritoneal fluid volume apparently influenced early reports which suggested that concentrations of peritoneal fluid prostaglandin levels were elevated in women with endometriosis (Drake *et al.* 1981; Dawood *et al.* 1984). Badaway *et al.* (1982), who corrected for the changes in fluid volume with the phases of the cycle, showed elevations in prostaglandins in the secretory phase only. In reviewing the prostaglandin studies, Schmidt (1985) concluded that further study is required before their role (if any) is fully understood. Thus it is not yet possible to establish a cause-and-effect relationship between prostaglandins and infertility in patients with minimal endometriosis.

Immunological disorders

Humoral antibodies to endometrial tissue have been identified in the serum of women with endometriosis (Mathur *et al.* 1982; Badaway *et al.* 1984*a*). It is suggested but not proven that these antibodies interfere with normal endometrial development, and hence with implantation.

The numbers and activity of peritoneal macrophages are increased in patients with endometriosis (Haney *et al.* 1981; Halme *et al.* 1984*b*). However, a similar finding has been noted in women without endometriosis (Olive *et al.* 1985; Koninckx *et al.* 1978). Whether macrophage activity represents a cause or an effect of endometriosis remains unclear.

Hormonal disturbances

Prolactin and gonadotrophin metabolism may be altered in patients with endometriosis. The evidence with respect to gonadotrophin function is scant. Cheesman *et al.* (1982) report that 26 to 29 patients with endometriosis showed evidence of not one but two peaks of LH release. Alper and Siebel (1986) were not able to confirm this finding.

Hirschowitz *et al.* (1978) and Hargrove and Abraham (1980) have demonstrated elevated prolactin levels in some women with endo-metriosis. Muse and Wilson (1982) showed an augmented prolactin response to thyrotropin-releasing hormone in 14 endometriosis patients when compared to controls. But this study was performed immediately before surgery; and Corenblum and Taylor (1981) have demonstrated that the apprehension preceding laparoscopy is suf-ficent to alter prolactin dynamics in an unpredictable fashion. It has not been shown that the elevation of prolactin in asymptomatic women is a cause of infertility (Glazener *et al.* 1987*a*).

THERAPEUTIC TRIALS

Data from two types of therapeutic trials can help to evaluate whether minimal and mild endometriosis cause infertility. In both types of trial, the pregnancy rate is the outcome of interest. One type compares women who have untreated minimal or mild endo-metriosis with those who have untreated unexplained infertility. The other evaluates treatment versus no treatment in women with minimal or mild endometriosis.

Forsey and Hull (1989) prospectively compared 31 couples with minimal endometriosis to 38 couples with unexplained infertility. The cumulative pregnancy rates after 24 months from the time of diagnostic laparoscopy were 25 per cent for the endometriosis group and 50 per cent for the unexplained infertility group. These data do not imply causality; whether the lower rate was due to the minimal endometriosis or to some undetectable coincidental factor remains unclear.

Turning to treatment versus no treatment, an early, non-randomized study (Schenken and Malinak 1982) of patients who either were treated surgically or were not treated demonstrated a 75 per cent pregnancy rate in both groups within 12 months of diagnosis. More recently, Chan and Collins (in press) have reviewed those studies which compared treated infertile women with untreated or placebo-treated controls. Five studies were identified which evaluated ovulation suppression with a steroid hormone derivative (Bayer *et al.* 1988; Hull *et al.* 1987; Levinson 1989; Telimaa 1988; and Thomas and Cooke 1987). In the analysis, the treatment effect was expressed as the odds of pregnancy with and without treatment. In the individual studies the odds ratios ranged from 0.6 to 1.3, none of which were significant (Table 7.1). The combined odds ratio was 0.9 (95 per cent CI 0.6 to 1.2), and this suggests that ovulation suppression therapy, which reduces the extent of visible endometriosis, does not improve fertility. Thus, although minimal and mild endometriosis seem likely to be related to a causal chain leading to infertility, direct treatment has not been demonstrated to improve fertility.

INVESTIGATION

The presence of endometriosis may be suggested by the history, although a history of infertility alone is sufficient to arouse suspicion, or by physical examination. A presumptive diagnosis and staging require laparoscopy, and the diagnosis is finally confirmed by histological evaluation of biopsy specimens. Attempts have been made to identify substances in the bloodstream which might act as peripheral markers for the disease. Non-invasive imaging techniques are being explored.

Table 7.1 *Effect of steroid hormone therapy on subsequent pregnancy rate*

Authors	Treatment group	Number of subjects pregnant/total		Odds ratio (95 per cent CI)*	*p* value for Mantel–Haenszel statistic
		Treated	Control		
Thomas and Cooke 1987	gestrinone	5/20	4/17	1.1 (0.2 to 6.3)	0.78
Bayer *et al.* 1988	danazol	13/37	17/36	0.6 (0.2 to 1.7)	0.42
Telimaa 1988	danazol	6/18	6/14	0.7 (0.1 to 3.5)	0.86
	MPA†	7/17	6/14	0.9 (0.2 to 5.0)	0.79
Levinson 1989	danazol	40/85	53/104	0.9 (0.5 to 1.6)	0.59
Hull *et al.* 1987	danazol	18/52	21/56	0.9 (0.4 to 2.1)	0.91
	MPA†	16/36	21/56	1.3 (0.5 to 3.4)	0.66
Combined odds ratio				0.9 (0.6 to 1.2)	0.54

* Breslow–Day test for homogeneity (6 df) = 1.86, *p* = 0.93
† MPA: medroxyprogesterone acetate

The timing of laparoscopy

Certain historical or physical findings suggestive of the presence of endometriosis would indicate earlier recourse to laparoscopy. These include chronic pelvic pain, severe dysmenorrhoea, deep dyspareunia, and abnormal uterine bleeding. Rectal pain, tenesmus, haematuria, and cyclic rectal bleeding should raise the index of suspicion. A family history of endometriosis in a first-degree relative would also justify such an approach (Simpson *et al.* 1980). The disease is more common in women who have never been pregnant, but can afflict women in any age or ethnic group. Primary infertility alone is not an indication for early laparoscopy.

At the time of bi-manual examination, findings of tenderness, nodularity, ovarian enlargement, fixed retroversion, and thickening of the recto-vaginal septum are highly suggestive that endometriosis is present and would warrant early endoscopic evaluation. If possible, laparoscopy should be performed a day or so before the expected onset of menstruation (Yuzpe *et al.* 1986). At this time, the lesions tend to be more prominent, and may be seen to be bleeding.

Appearance of lesions

Lesions observed laparoscopically cover a spectrum from the classical 'gunpowder burn' of 2–5 mm in size to total pelvic disorganization, with dense adhesions and large intra-ovarian chocolate cysts. Peritoneal defects may represent old lesions. Enlarged ovaries which are adherent one to the other, the so-called 'kissing ovaries', are pathognomonic. The prevalence of visible endometriosis in women with infertility varies from 1 to 21 per cent.

The gold standard of diagnosis is histological evaluation of biopsy specimens, more particularly as increasing evidence is accumulating that areas of peritoneum which do not have the classical appearances of endometriosis may in fact contain histologically typical lesions.

Jansen and Russell (1986) reviewed 137 biopsies taken from peritoneal lesions which did not have the classical appearance of endometriosis. Typical endometrial glands and stroma were seen in 73 (53 per cent). Martin *et al.* (1989) increased the rate of diagnosis from 42 per cent to 72 per cent by using the magnifying capabilities of the laparoscopic telescope to identify non-typical areas from which peritoneal biopsies were taken. Nisolle *et al.* (1990) performed laparoscopy in 118 patients complaining of infertility: 86 were diagnosed laparoscopically as suffering from endometriosis. Ninety-three per cent of biopsies taken from typical lesions were histologically positive. Thirteen per cent of biopsies taken from apparently healthy peritoneum in the patients were also positive. In the 32 women who were apparently disease-free, histological evidence of endometriosis was detected in 6 per cent.

These microscopic findings in apparently healthy peritoneum are intriguing; but the caveat of Murphy *et al.* (1989) cannot be reiterated too strongly. Until the prevalence of these lesions among fertile women is known, it is improper to assume an association with infertility.

Non-invasive tests

The search for a non-invasive marker for the presence of endometriosis has largely focused on CA-125, a membrane antigen. Elevated levels were detected in the serum of 80 per cent of women with ovarian cancer and 49 per cent of women with Stage III or IV endometriosis (Barbieri 1986). The test is not practical for the assessment of infertile women. Takahashi *et al.* (1990) measured CA-125 in menstrual blood of women with endometriosis. Overall, the sensitivity of the test was 66 per cent, 60 per cent for Stages I, II, and III, and 72 per cent for Stage IV. While apparently more accurate than serum values, this test still is not sufficiently specific to be used effectively. Attempts to use serum complement levels as a marker have likewise been unsuccessful (Badawy *et al.* 1984*a*). Ultrasound may be helpful in assessing ovarian cyst formation, but is unable to identify Stage I and Stage II lesions.

CONCLUSIONS

The diagnosis and staging of endometriosis remains a function of laparoscopy and histological evaluation of biopsy specimens.

Accepting that moderate (Stage III) and severe (Stage IV) endo-metriosis cause infertility is not difficult. It is virtually impossible to draw conclusions about how minimal (Stage I) and mild (Stage II) endometriosis relate to infertility. As their incidence in a normal population is unknown, all that can be said is that minimal and mild endometriosis are observed in women with infertility.

No satisfactory mechanism has been described to explain how Stage I or Stage II endometriosis could cause infertility. Conception rates are, however, lower than in unexplained fertility (Forsey and Hull 1989). Treatment does not improve fertility. The question 'Does minimal or mild endometriosis cause infertility, or does childlessness due to some unidentifiable cause simply permit the lesions to develop?' cannot yet be answered.

Definition

Stage III or Stage IV endometriosis provides an explanation for infertility. Because fertility is reduced in patients with Stage I and Stage II endometriosis, the finding of such lesions precludes a diagnosis of unexplained infertility.

---

8 Immunological phenomena

An immune response may be mounted against spermatozoa in both the male and the female, and against the oocyte in the female. Detection of an immunological error might constitute an explanation for infertility. This chapter will briefly review basic immunological physiology, and describe the influence of the immune system on reproduction. The investigations and their applicability to the clinical situation will then be described.

BASIC IMMUNOLOGY

The immune system is designed to recognize foreign material and to mount a defensive response. This defensive response may be humoral, that is, by the elaboration of antibodies aimed against the foreign material (antigen). A cellular response also operates, whereby cells either engulf the foreign material, or elaborate chemicals which may affect the action of other cells, or directly alter the foreign material.

The system is complex. The antigenic make-up of an individual is coded on chromosome number six. The antigen region is described as the major histocompatibility complex. The best-understood system within this complex contains the human leukocyte antigens (HLA), which are critical for tissue typing in organ transplantation. Four transplantation antigens are described. A, B, and C are present in the plasma membranes of most cells. DR is present in specialized cells only.

While under certain conditions mast cells and eosinophils may be involved in the immune response, the most important cellular components are the lymphocytes and macrophages. Three major families of lymphocytes are identified: T (thymus) cells, responsible for the cell-mediated response; B (bursa) cells, responsible for antibody production; and natural killer (NK) cells.

The T cells act as immunological watchdogs, and produce cellular mediators which may stimulate macrophages and B cells. Two major subpopulations of T cells exist: helper cells, which augment, and suppressor cells, which inhibit the immune response. B cells are responsible for antibody production. The NK cells, which act without prior exposure to lyse invading cells, are the body's first line of defence.

Macrophages primarily function to engulf foreign material. They may be fixed in specific parts of the body or may be migratory. They are triggered to act by lymphokines and other mediators released by T-lymphocytes.

The second component of the immune response is humoral. Antibodies, in the form of immunoglobulins, are produced in response to an antigenic stimulus. These may bind to and neutralize the antigen or act through the complement system.

Five classes of immunoglobulins (Igs) are described in the human: IgG, IgA, IgM, IgD, and IgE. The predominant Ig in serum is IgG. Locally produced antibodies tend to be IgA.

When an antigen enters the system, if receptors are present on the B-cell membrane, the antigen is bound and stimulates the B-cell to produce the necessary specific immunoglobulin. This process may be augmented by the presence of T helper cells. Many antigens are not initially recognized by the B cells until they have first been processed by phagocytic antigen processing cells (APCs). The antigen is bound to the surface of the APC. This binding allows the helper cell to recognize the foreign protein. The helper cell modifies the B cells so that they also may recognize the antigen, proliferate, and begin antibody (immunoglobulin) production (Bronson 1990). Subsequent exposure to the antigen may activate the B cell directly.

Much of the antibody response is mediated through the complement system. When activated, a cascade of more than 20 plasma proteins occurs, finally resulting in the formation of a membrane attack complex (MAC). The MAC lyses cellular membranes. In addition, complement is leukotactic, and attracts polymorphonuclear leukocytes to the affected area.

The proteins of the zona pellucida are not immunologically

foreign to the woman. Nevertheless, antibodies directed against the zona pellucida have been demonstrated in women complaining of infertility (Bousquet *et al.* 1982). Little is known of the clinical importance of such antibodies. Spermatozoa are, however, immunologically foreign for the female, and hence might act as antigens to provoke a potential clinical response. Because many of the antigens on the spermatozoa are elaborated after the embryological period during which immunological recognition of self is imprinted, spermatozoa can be a stimulus to antibody production if they gain access to the male system. Thus anti-sperm antibodies in the male could be of clinical significance.

REPRODUCTIVE IMMUNOLOGY

Immunology of semen

Semen possesses both antigenic and immunosuppressive properties (Alexander and Anderson 1987).

The antigens of the spermatozoa are acquired gradually as the sperm cell matures. Antigenic sites have been mapped on the acrosome, post-acrosome, equatorial region, mid-piece, tail, and tip of the tail (Alexander and Anderson 1987). While most are situated on the surface, some are only exposed after the outer membranes of the acrosome have broken down. Sperm antigens can also be identified in the embryo (Solter and Schachner 1976), the ovary (Menge and Fleming 1978), and the placenta (Berkowitz *et al.* 1985).

Fortunately, the major histo-compatibility antigens, which might provoke a massive response by the female, are not expressed on the spermatozoa (Anderson *et al.* 1982).

The acquisition of sperm antigens occurs as the sperm cells mature, an event which begins at puberty, long after tolerance for self-antigens was established (Bronson 1990). Why then, do these late-appearing antigens normally fail to provoke an immune response in the adult male? Spermatozoa are produced in the tests, and an effective blood–testes barrier exists within the seminiferous tubules. This barrier prevents spermatic material from entering the circulatory system, and prevents lymphocytes, immunoglobulins, and complement from entering the testes (Gilula *et al.* 1976).

Thus, under normal circumstances, the spermatozoal antigens are effectively sequestered from the body's system of recognition. The blood—testes barrier in the rest of the ejaculatory system, while effective under normal conditions, can be breached during infection or traumatic (including post-vasectomy) episodes (Alexander and Anderson 1979; Mancini *et al.* 1965). If such a breach occurs, anti-sperm antibodies may be formed.

In addition to the blood—testes barrier, local immuno-regulatory events inhibit the formation of antibodies to spermatozoa. Suppressor cells, which prevent antibody formation by the B-cells, may be activated within the testis. Suppressor lymphocytes are found in the epididymis (Ritchie *et al.* 1984).

Seminal plasma inhibits T-cells, B-cells, natural killer cells, macrophages, polymorphonuclear leukocytes, and the actions of complement. Thus an extensive system of checks and balances is in place, the function of which is to prevent auto-immunity, both humoral and cellular, from developing in the adult male.

This system can break down. Anti-sperm antibodies may be detected in the sera of male subjects (Rumke and Hellinga 1959). Immunoglobulins can be detected on the sperm surface (Haas and Cunningham 1984). IgG antibodies, which are primarily a prostatic transudate (Rumke 1974), IgA antibodies, which are locally produced (Ayvaliotis *et al.* 1985), and complement components (Husted and Hjort 1975) have been detected in the seminal plasma.

The number of lymphocytes and activated macrophages is increased in the seminal plasma of some infertile male partners when compared to fertile controls, which suggested that cell-mediated as well as humoral mechanisms may become activated in such males (Anderson and Hill 1988). Lymphokines and monokines released by these cells can inhibit spermatic function (Maruyama *et al.* 1985).

Immune response to spermatozoa in the female

Once spermatozoa are deposited in the female genital tract, their surface antibodies are exposed to the female immune system. The genital tract is immunologically competent. IgG and IgA are present throughout the system, and are detectable in the vaginal secretions; the majority of the IgA is secreted locally (Chodirker and

Tomasi 1963). In cervical mucus, their concentrations fluctuate between the follicular phase (high) and mid-cycle (low) (Schumacher 1980). This pattern is reversed in the uterine secretions, where the levels are higher at mid-cycle (Bronson 1990). IgG and IgA have also been identified in tubal fluid (Lippes *et al.* 1972).

Anti-sperm antibodies found in uterine or tubal fluid are produced locally (IgA), and do not reflect levels found in the serum (Bronson 1990). Those found in peritoneal fluid are simply transudates of serum immunoglobulins. In cervical mucus, anti-sperm antibodies may be transudates or secreted locally.

Given the competence of the female immune system, why do not all women produce anti-sperm antibodies? It is probable that the immuno-suppressive factors found in the seminal plasma and described earlier in this chapter play a significant role (Bronson 1990).

How might an immune response against spermatic antigens interfere with fertility? It is probable that, unless sperm antibodies can gain access to the sperm cells, they are not capable of affecting fertility. Those that can gain access to spermatozoa may inhibit fertility by interfering with sperm movement or sperm function.

Antibodies could impair sperm motility and function by causing agglutination, reduced or total loss of motility, impaired cervical-mucus penetration, and inefficient sperm–egg fusion (Alexander and Anderson 1987). Fertilization could be impaired by sperm antibody bound to acrosin, a sperm enzyme which is essential to sperm–egg interactions. Howe *et al.* (1991) found, however, that only 30 per cent of 27 infertile women with sperm antibody had acrosin-specific binding, and their fertility was similar to that of the 70 per cent with no specific binding. Also, sperm-immobilizing antibodies appear to bind specific sperm-surface glycoprotein components that may be involved in sperm–zona binding (Tsuji *et al.* 1988); but a correlation with fertility in untreated patients has not yet been reported (Kobayashi *et al.* 1990). Furthermore, Bronson *et al.* (1982) have shown that antibody bound to the sperm head inhibited zona-binding in experiments using non-viable human oocytes. The same antibodies promoted penetration of zona-free hamster oocytes, thus suggesting that the site of action of the antibodies on spermatozoa is at the zona.

The cellular immune response may impair fertility through

enhanced phagocytosis of sperm or through pre- or post-implantation loss of the embryo. Cell-mediated immunity to spermatozoa and antibodies directed against the oocyte are among the potential processes that could be responsible; but such disorders cannot as yet be detected or combatted in clinical practice. The greatest potential for clinical application is in the study of antibody directed against spermatozoa. The following section will discuss the investigation and clinical relevance of anti-sperm antibody.

CLINICAL RELEVANCE OF ANTI-SPERM ANTIBODIES

As with other investigations, attempts to detect the presence of anti-sperm antibodies either can be made in every couple or can be applied selectively only to those couples who are apparently at higher risk. Such discriminatory use of an investigation presupposes that clues can be detected from the history, from physical examination, or from less specific screening tests. With respect to anti-sperm antibodies, no historical clues or physical findings are of value in the female partner. Given the known aetiological significance of infection and trauma in the male, such findings would warrant further investigation. Routine semen analysis may reveal agglutination or aggregation of the spermatozoa. While aggregation may be non-specific, true agglutination is usually antibody-mediated (Mortimer 1985a). Because antibodies can impair sperm motility, if either phenomenon is noted further immunological investigations may be warranted. Poor sperm penetration of cervical mucus, particularly if the 'shaking' phenomenon is noted during the SCMC test, is suggestive of the presence of anti-sperm antibody. It has further been suggested that a search should be made for anti-sperm antibody in all couples in whom the routine diagnostic procedures for infertility have failed to reveal an explanation (Bronson 1990). It may also be, however, that the correlations with clinical results and outcomes do not justify such pursuits.

While it is simple to suggest that evidence of the presence of anti-sperm antibodies should be sought, the methods available for their detection are varied and complex. Furthermore, the appropriate site of antibody presence (serum, semen, spermatozoa, cervical mucus) to be investigated is unclear. The succeeding sections will describe the tests available, their correlation with one another, the correlations between antibody present in the various physiological compartments, and the correlation between anti-sperm antibodies and conventional tests of sperm function. Finally, and most importantly, the correlation between anti-sperm antibody results and pregnancy will be discussed.

Tests of anti-sperm antibodies

Because of the different types of antibody and the different mechanisms (agglutination of sperm, impairment of sperm motility, impairment of cervical-mucus penetration, and reduction of fertilization ability) whereby they may impair fertility, it is unlikely that any single test would suffice.

Originally bio-assays using donor semen were used to detect antibody in sera, and depended on the observation of agglutination (Franklin and Dukes 1964) or immobilization (Isojima *et al.* 1972) of the spermatozoa. These tests are frequently referred to as the serum agglutination test (SAT) and the serum immobilizing test (SIT). The presence of non-specific agglutination and the subsequently recognized need to perform certain assays in diluted semen have reduced the validity of some early studies which used these assays (Rose *et al.* 1976; Bronson 1990).

Newer techniques have been developed to detect specific immunoglobulins. The mixed agglutination reaction (MAR) uses red blood cells sensitized to anti-rhesus IgG (Jager *et al.* 1978). A drop of serum and rabbit anti-human IgG are mixed. If anti-sperm antibody is present on the spermatozoa, both the spermatozoa and the red blood cells agglutinate, an observable phenomenon which can be quantified with the use of dilutions.

Both modifications of the radio-labelled Coombs' antiglobulin test have also been used to measure plasma IgG to sperm (the radio-labelled antiglobulin test (RA) (Haas *et al.* 1980). The assay appears to detect both surface and internal sperm antigen (Haas *et al.* 1991).

Both enzyme-linked immuno-absorbent assay (ELISA) (Hjort *et al.* 1985) and a method using antibodies against human immunoglobulins coated on micro-titre wells (Hancock and Faruki 1984) can be used as screening tests. The ELISA methods are positive in 7 to 40 per cent of infertile women; but they are also positive in a correspondingly high percentage of fertile women (Hjort *et al.* 1985).

Polyacrylamide spheres can be covalently linked to rabbit anti-human immunoglobulins: the immunobead test (IB) (Bronson *et al.* 1981; Clarke *et al.* 1985*a*). Beads can be linked with IgG, IgA, and IgM antibodies, and thus can identify the specific immunoglobulin present on the spermatozoa. Furthermore, the specific site of bead-binding on the spermatozoa indicates where the antibody is bound to the spermatozoa. The assay can be performed on any body fluid or secretion when spermatozoa known to be antibody-free are first exposed to the material under scrutiny and then to the immuno-beads (Bronson *et al.* 1982). Intra-assay variability appears to be low, but inter-assay variability is higher, because of the differences in the individual sperm samples (Franco *et al.* 1987).

Correlation of different tests and frequency of anti-sperm antibody presence

The classical methods of identifying the presence of antibody generally correlate well with techniques which identify the presence of specific immunoglobulins (Table 8.1). Values of Kappa, which express agreement between the methods, are considerably greater than the agreement to be expected by chance alone. The agreement observed is independent of the biological milieu (serum, semen, or cervical mucus). The weighted Kappa values were highest in reports on immunobead tests (0.87 ± 0.02); weighted Kappa was 0.65 ± 0.03 in ELISA reports and 0.62 ± 0.03 in MAR reports. The discrepancies are readily explained as those variations that occur when the concentration of any substance is estimated by different methods.

Because the published reports suggest that the various tests for the presence of antibody are highly correlated, it was judged reasonable to pool the results of studies based on different methods that estimate the frequency of anti-sperm antibody in men and women.

Among male infertile partners the frequency of anti-sperm antibody ranges in the serum from 1 to 28 per cent; in the aggregate

Table 8.1 *Reported agreement between functional assays for sperm antibody in serum and immunoglobulin-specific assays in serum, semen, and cervical mucus*

Functional assay	Specific assays Locus	Number of subjects	Kappa value	Specific immunoglobulin assay*	Authors
Agglutinating antibody	serum	75	0.31	MAR G	Cimino *et al.* 1986
		83	0.44	RA G	Haas *et al.* 1980
		292	0.88	ELISA	Lynch *et al.* 1986
		70	0.40	ELISA GM	Wolff and Schill 1985
		46	0.35	ELISA	Zanchetta *et al.* 1982
	semen	178	0.87	MAR G	Adeghe *et al.* 1986
		178	0.98	IB G	Adeghe *et al.* 1986
		186	0.67	ELISA G	Alexander and Bearwood 1984
		299	0.73	MAR G	Francavilla *et al.* 1984
		202	0.90	IB GA	Jennings *et al.* 1985
		537	0.54	MAR GA	Meinertz and Hjort 1986
Immobilizing antibody	mucus	83	0.69	IB A	Clarke *et al.* 1984
	serum	75	0.49	MAR G	Cimino *et al.* 1986
	semen	186	0.41	ELISA G	Alexander and Bearwood 1984
		135	0.82	IB G	Clarke *et al.* 1985*a*
		138	0.77	IB A	Clarke *et al.* 1985*a*
		202	0.93	IB GA	Jennings *et al.* 1985

* Specific immunoglobulin assays: ELISA, enzyme-linked immunosorbent assay; IB, immunobead assay; MAR, mixed antiglobulin reaction test; RA, radio-labelled anti-globulin test. Immunoglobulins: A, G, M.

Table 8.2 *Frequency of sperm antibody in various groups of men*

Diagnostic category	Number of assays	Number positive	Percentage positive (range)	Weighted mean (per cent)
Infertility, diagnosis unspecified*	7932	708	1 to 29	8.9
Unexplained infertility†	415	48	6 to 21	11.6
Proven fertility‡	182	5	2 to 8	2.8

References

* Ansbacher *et al*. 1973; Badawy *et al*. 1984*b*; Baker *et al*. 1983; Eggert-Kruse *et al*. 1989*a*; Francavilla *et al*. 1984; Haas *et al*. 1983; Hanafiah *et al*. 1972; Handelsman *et al*. 1983; Hargreave 1982; Ingerslev and Ingerslev 1980; Lynch *et al*. 1986; Menge *et al*. 1982; Moghissi *et al*. 1980; Rumke and Hellinga 1959; Schoenfeld *et al*. 1976; Telang *et al*. 1978; Upadhyaya *et al*. 1984; Wolff and Schill 1985; Zanchetta *et al*. 1982.

† Bronson *et al*. 1985; Hanafiah *et al*. 1972; Rodgers-Neame *et al*. 1986.

‡ Bronson *et al*. 1985; Upadhyaya *et al*. 1984.

published data, the frequency is similar in unexplained infertility and other infertility diagnostic categories, and in both cases it is 3 to 4 times higher than in fertile men (Table 8.2).

The frequency of anti-sperm antibody on the sperm surface is of the order of 7 to 15 per cent, and in seminal fluid from 1 to 7 per cent (Collins 1988). Clarke *et al*. (1985*a*) compared the presence of antibody in the serum and semen in 845 infertile men. Antibody was detected in the serum but not on the spermatozoa, where it is believed any deleterious effect must be mediated, in 20 per cent of patients; and in 14 per cent antibody was bound to spermatozoa but was not present in the serum.

Among female partners the frequency of anti-sperm antibody ranges in serum from 1 to 22 per cent, and in cervical mucus from 5 to 31 per cent (Collins 1988). The reported frequency in serum is essentially similar in women with otherwise explained infertility and those whose infertility is unexplained. Neither frequency is materially higher than the frequency among fertile women (Table 8.3).

Correlation between other assessments of fertility and anti-sperm antibodies

Correlations between independent assessments of fertility status and anti-sperm antibody might suggest by which mechanisms the detri-

Table 8.3 *Frequency of sperm antibody in various groups of women*

Diagnostic category	Number of assays	Number positive	Percentage positive (range)	Weighted mean (per cent)
Infertility, diagnosis unspecified*	4847	455	1 to 22	9.4
Unexplained infertility†	672	59	6 to 12	8.8
Proven fertility‡	119	5	0 to 10	4.2

References

* Ansbacher *et al.* 1973; Badawy *et al.* 1984*b*; Chen and Jones 1981; Eggert-Kruse *et al.* 1989*a*; Hanafiah *et al.* 1972; Hargreave 1982; Ingerslev and Ingerslev 1980; Menge *et al.* 1982; Moghissi *et al.* 1980; Rumke and Hellinga 1959; Schoenfeld *et al.* 1976; Telang *et al.* 1978.

† Bronson *et al.* 1985; Chen and Jones 1981; Hanafiah *et al.* 1972; Ingerslev and Ingerslev 1980; Rodgers-Neame *et al.* 1986; Witkin *et al.* 1984.

‡ Bronson *et al.* 1985; Witkin *et al.* 1984.

mental effects are mediated. Antibody present in the ejaculate may interfere with sperm motility; sperm antibody is more frequent in men with low sperm motility (34 per cent) than in men with normal motility (5 per cent) (Barratt *et al.* 1989*b*). Nevertheless, correlations with seminal characteristics are not uniform (Eggert-Kruse *et al.* 1989*a*). This section will discuss in greater detail the association between anti-sperm antibody presence and both sperm–cervical-mucus tests and sperm–oocyte interaction.

Sperm–cervical-mucus tests

The postcoital test

Immunoglobulins bound to the sperm surface appear to inhibit the ability of sperm to penetrate cervical mucus (Jager *et al.* 1984). Thus, the postcoital test should correlate with anti-sperm antibody presence, and might serve as a screening test.

Postcoital test results do not accurately predict anti-sperm antibody presence in either the female partner's serum or the male partner's serum (Table 8.4). The Kappa values are less than 0.40 in all but one report, suggesting that the observed agreement is little better than might occur by chance. As a screening test for anti-sperm antibody, the postcoital test is not sufficiently sensitive;

Table 8.4 *Utility of the postcoital test as a screening test for anti-sperm antibody presence*

Milieu	Number of subjects	Sensitivity (per cent)	Specificity (per cent)	Kappa value	Authors
Female partner's serum					
	53	80	29	0.02	Badawy *et al.* 1984*b*
	235	23	86	0.09	Eggert-Kruse *et al.* 1989*a*
	82	13	89	0.02	Friberg 1981*a*
	293	74	59	0.33	Mathur *et al.* 1984
	84	62	61	0.13	Moghissi *et al.* 1980
	28	38	25	−0.17	Pretorius and Franken 1989
	24	50	55	0.01	Soffer *et al.* 1976
	127	64	80	0.41	Telang *et al.* 1978
Male partner's serum					
	53	70	28	−0.01	Badawy *et al.* 1984*b*
	233	17	88	0.05	Eggert-Kruse *et al.* 1989*a*
	93	70	89	0.55	Friberg 1981*b*
	41	100	49	0.16	Haas *et al.* 1983
	293	75	64	0.33	Mathur *et al.* 1984
	75	75	61	0.08	Moghissi *et al.* 1980
	28	79	75	0.38	Pretorius and Franken 1989
	123	20	69	−0.07	Telang *et al.* 1978
Cervical mucus					
	42	91	24	0.16	Dor *et al.* 1977
	82	82	61	0.21	Moghissi *et al.* 1980
	24	100	72	0.57	Soffer *et al.* 1976
	45	64	71	0.33	Telang *et al.* 1978
Sperm surface					
	34	67	100	0.68	Bronson *et al.* 1984
	71	92	44	0.31	Haas *et al.* 1983

screening tests should possess the ability to identify a high proportion of subjects with possible antibody presence, even if that is ruled out by the more accurate confirmatory test (in this case the antibody assay). With respect to cervical-mucus and sperm-surface antibodies, the screening value of the postcoital test was generally no better, although two studies did achieve Kappa values greater than 0.50 (Bronson *et al.* 1984; Soffer *et al.* 1976).

Given the recognized difficulties of the postcoital test, attempts have been made to correlate the findings of antibody presence with *in vitro* tests of mucus penetration by sperm. Impaired mucus penetration might reflect more directly the antibody activity in cervical mucus or on the sperm surface rather than antibody activity in serum. The shaking phenomenon observed in the sperm–cervical-mucus contact test appears to be due to secretory IgA antibodies, but high titres occur in less than 1 per cent of infertile women (Jager *et al.* 1977; Jager *et al.* 1984). One retrospective study has indicated that sperm shaking and reduced cervical-mucus penetration are correlated, but whether the observed lower pregnancy rates are related to the presence of anti-sperm antibody has not been confirmed (Menge *et al.* 1982). Another prospective study has failed to confirm an association between *in vitro* mucus-penetration results and anti-sperm antibody presence in either partner (Eggert-Kruse *et al.* 1989*b*).

The lack of consistency in the correlation between anti-sperm antibody presence and sperm motility in cervical mucus does not justify the use of either postcoital tests or *in vitro* mucus-penetration tests as screening tests on the basis of present knowledge.

Sperm–oocyte interaction

The results of the zona-free hamster assay, human zona-binding studies, and data from human *in vitro* fertilization programmes can be correlated with anti-sperm antibody status. Spermatozoa which can penetrate hamster oocytes lose this ability when incubated with sperm-agglutinating antibodies. Disagglutination and restoration of penetrating ability can be effected using proteolytic enzymes (Pattinson *et al.* 1990). Antibody bound to the sperm head can inhibit binding to human zonae, but does not prevent the ability to penetrate zona-free hamster oocytes, thus indicating that such antibodies may inhibit the sperm binding to the zona pellucida. Thus it is not surprising that the penetration of zona-free hamster eggs was diminished but not abolished by the presence of high levels of antibody (Abdel-Latif *et al.* 1986; Alexander 1984; Haas 1985).

With respect to human *in vitro* fertilization, anti-sperm antibody presence in male serum, female serum, or cervical mucus may reduce fertilization rates (Ackerman *et al.* 1984; Clarke *et al.* 1986; Yovich *et al.* 1984). Others have not been able to demonstate any influence of the presence of antibody upon fertilization or pregnancy rates (Ausmanas *et al.* 1986). In one study, although fertilization rates were reduced, the pregnancy rate did not appear to be influenced by the presence of anti-sperm antibody (Mandelbaum *et al.* 1987).

Much of the information on the correlation between anti-sperm antibody and other evaluations of fertile status is conflicting or unclear. The fundamental question remains: does the presence of anti-sperm antibody reduce the likelihood of pregnancy?

Anti-sperm antibody presence and fertility

Although a correlation between anti-sperm antibody presence and pregnancy would be a key element in any argument that infertility could be caused by immune errors, very few studies have addressed this question, and even fewer have evaluated antibody presence or absence among fully investigated couples with unexplained infertility.

Table 8.5 summarizes studies which evaluate antibody presence in the male or the female partner with respect to conception during follow-up. Excluded are studies in which antibody in either partner defined the 'antibody present' group (Hanafiah *et al.* 1972; Mathur *et al.* 1981; Mathur *et al.* 1984). Also excluded are studies in which all subjects were antibody-positive, even though some subjects with lower titres or other characteristics served as controls (Ayvaliotis *et al.* 1985; Howe *et al.* 1991; Rumke 1974; Rumke *et al.* 1984).

The studies included in the table have several design short-comings: retrospective assembly with questionnaire follow-up (Ansbacher *et al.* 1973; Menge *et al.* 1982); treatment confounding (Ansbacher *et al.* 1973; Baker *et al.* 1983); and the use of a singular antibody assay method (Blumenfeld *et al.* 1986). In one study of male partners, a history of vasectomy reversal was reported for 17 of 72 antibody-positive men, and none of 753 antibody-negative controls (Baker *et al.* 1983).

Anti-sperm antibody in the female partner's serum was associated with significantly lower fertility in only one study (Menge *et al.* 1982) (Table 8.5). This retrospective study with questionnaire-based follow-up had a very low odds ratio (0.09; 95 per cent CI:

Table 8.5 *Sperm antibody presence and fertility*

Milieu	Number of subjects	Pregnancy rate with 95 per cent confidence interval		Odds ratio*	Authors
		Antibody absent	Antibody present		
Female partner's serum					
	185	52 ± 8	42 ± 19	0.7	Ansbacher *et al.* 1973
	110	10 ± 6	0 ± 0	0.4	Blumenfeld *et al.* 1986
	235	28 ± 6	21 ± 12	0.7	Eggert-Kruse *et al.* 1989*a*
	326	40 ± 5	53 ± 22	1.7	Ingerslev and Ingerslev 1980
	376	46 ± 6	7 ± 5	0.1	Menge *et al.* 1982
Male partner's serum					
	172	52 ± 8	31 ± 25	0.4	Ansbacher *et al.* 1973
	825	30 ± 3	8 ± 6	0.2	Baker *et al.* 1983
	233	26 ± 6	35 ± 16	1.6	Eggert-Kruse *et al.* 1989*a*
	376	43 ± 6	19 ± 8	0.3	Menge *et al.* 1982

* Relative probability of pregnancy if antibody is present

0.03, 0.21). Considering only the three prospective studies in this Table, however, which included 671 subjects, the combined odds ratio was 0.9 (95 per cent CI: 0.5, 1.6), indicating that on the best evidence available there is the possibility of a small but insignificant reduction in conception rates associated with detectable levels of anti-sperm antibody (Blumenfeld *et al.* 1986; Eggert-Kruse *et al.* 1989*a*; Ingerslev and Ingerslev 1980).

With respect to male partners, anti-sperm antibody presence in serum was associated with a significantly lower pregnancy rate in two of four studies (Baker *et al.* 1983; Menge *et al.* 1982). In the only male study which was prospective and free from confounding by treatment and vasectomy reversal, the pregnancy rate was slightly higher in the antibody-present cohort (Eggert-Kruse *et al.* 1989*a*).

Two studies have evaluated immobilizing antibodies in cervical mucus among couples with unexplained infertility. The pregnancy rate in the presence of antibody was 19 per cent higher (Chen and Jones 1981) and 23 per cent lower (Menge *et al.* 1982) than the rates in the antibody-negative comparison couples.

Because antibody to spermatozoa is not a common finding in

couples with unexplained infertility, large prospective studies based on newer validated assay methods are needed among untreated couples to evaluate whether sperm antibody is a cause of infertility. Until these studies have been conducted, and until some of the many possible mechanisms have been defined, any link between sperm antibody presence and impaired conception must be considered hypothetical.

SUMMARY

The immunology of human reproduction is complex. With respect to infertility, the most studied immune mechanism is the presence and function of anti-sperm antibodies. Although in the male an association with infertility has been shown, antibody presence is neither consistent from time to time in the individual nor exclusive to the infertile state. The association with infertility could be explained by means of a hypothesis whereby antibodies to one or more sperm antigens interfere with one or more mechanisms of reproduction. This hypothesis has not been proved.

Other hypotheses are also plausible. Anti-sperm antibody synthesis in either partner could be a normal response to sperm antigen. This seems unlikely in the male partner, where anti-sperm antibodies are more likely after a history of surgery, trauma, or infection. In the female partner, however, none of the clinical data are inconsistent with a normal function for anti-sperm antibody.

Also plausible is the hypothesis that anti-sperm antibody presence in either partner is a reaction to errors in spermatogenesis, sperm transport systems, or sperm function. In this hypothesis it is the underlying error that is primarily responsible for the infertile state and its diversity. In this case, the presence of anti-sperm antibody would be no more than a marker for the hidden defect, and would not necessarily relate to the severity of the defect.

Given the clinical uncertainty that arises from these and other possible explanations for the association between anti-sperm antibody and infertility, it would be premature to require an assessment of anti-sperm antibody status in either partner as a pre-requisite to the diagnosis of unexplained infertility.

Definition of infertility with respect to immunological factors

While immunological events may well be responsible for infertility, current understanding does not permit an explanation based on clinical testing. The presence of antibody to sperm does not refute the diagnosis of unexplained infertility.

9 Infective agents

Severe damage to the fallopian tubes or male ejaculatory system leading to infertility can be caused by the sequelae of infection by specific micro-organisms, including *Neisseria gonorrhoeae*, *Mycobacterium tuberculosis*, and *Chlamydia trachomatis*. In the absence of such overt damage, can infertility be explained by detecting evidence of a specific micro-organism in either partner? Three particular organisms have been of recent interest—the *Mycoplasmas*, *Ureaplasma urealyticum*, and *Chlamydia trachomatis*.

MYCOPLASMA HOMINIS AND UREAPLASMA UREALYTICUM

The *Mycoplasmas* were first identified in 1937 (Dienes and Edsall 1937). The genus *Mycoplasma* encompasses more than 60 species. The species *Ureaplasma urealyticum*, once called T-mycoplasma, has been accorded distinct status due to its ability to hydrolyse urea (Styler and Shapiro 1985). These organisms have a trilaminar cell membrane and no cell wall, and contain both RNA and DNA. They are the size of large viruses, and multiple serotypes of both *M. hominis* and *U. urealyticum* have been identified (Styler and Shapiro 1985). They are rarely found in the uterus and tubes of healthy women (Taylor-Robinson and McCormack 1979). The most frequently evaluated sites in the investigation of infertility are the semen and cervical mucus. There is no evidence that the presence of *U. urealyticum* in cervical mucus or semen inhibits sperm motility or viability (Gump *et al.* 1984). Although degenerative changes can be shown in the human fallopian tube in tissue culture in the presence of *M. hominis* (Mardh *et al.* 1976), these effects have not been reported *in vivo* (Styler and Shapiro 1985). A ciliostatic effect of *U.*

urealyticum has been noted in bovine oviduct in tissue culture (Stalheim *et al.* 1976); but this effect cannot be replicated in the human fallopian tube.

Penetration of the zona-free hamster egg by human sperm is altered if sperm samples are exposed to either *M. hominis* or *U. urealyticum* (Busolo and Zanchetta 1985). This effect differed depending upon the serotype of the *Ureaplasma* species. Fifty-one per cent of oocytes were penetrated by sperm incubated with Type 1—a rate not different from that of controls. Only 6 per cent were penetrated when serotype 4 was investigated.

As clear evidence of a mechanism could not be demonstrated whereby these organisms might cause infertility, it was hoped that epidemiological studies or therapeutic trials might provide some insight. Epidemiological studies are confounded by the high prevalence of the organisms in the general population. *U. urealyticum* has been found in the cervical mucus of 23 per cent (Gnarpe and Friberg 1972) to 68 per cent (Khatamee and Decker 1978) of pregnant women.

The majority of studies comparing infertile women with fertile controls has failed to demonstrate significant differences in the prevalence of either *Mycoplasma* or *Ureaplasma* (Styler and Shapiro 1985). Treatment trials using doxycycline or erythromycin to eradicate these organisms have been similarly disappointing (Styler and Shapiro 1985). It would appear that a causative role in infertility for *M. hominis* and *U. urealyticum* remains unproven.

CHLAMYDIA TRACHOMATIS

Chlamydia trachomatis is an obligate intracellular parasite. It has a cell wall which is similar in structure to that of the Gram-negative bacteria. It contains both RNA and DNA. Because of its intracellular location, it can only be grown in tissue culture. Properly performed tissue culture has a sensitivity of 80–90 per cent and a specificity of 100 per cent (Monif 1990). Unfortunately, tissue culture is extremely expensive.

Alternative approaches to identifying the presence of the organism include direct smear fluorescent antibody testing, enzyme-linked immuno-assay, and the examination of the serum for IgG and IgM antichlamydial antibodies.

The direct smear fluorescent antibody test has a sensitivity greater than 90 per cent and a specificity greater than 98 per cent (Monif 1990). Micro-immunofluorescence is a more sensitive test than the classical complement fixation method for the detection of humoral antibodies.

C. trachomatis is the most frequently sexually transmitted microorganism (Westrom 1980). It can cause severe anatomical disruption to the fallopian tubes (Moore *et al.* 1982; Kane *et al.* 1984). Whether or not the presence of the organism in the genital tract of women in whom the tubes are anatomically normal, or in the semen or genital tract of men, causes infertility is unclear. Using serum antibody titres, Eggert-Kruse *et al.* (1990) screened 491 infertile male partners. No significant correlation was noted with semen analysis or other assessments of spermatic function and positive or negative antibody titres. They concluded that *C. trachomatis* does not reduce sperm functional capacity. This study also failed to reveal a cause-and-effect relationship between *C. trachomatis* and the formation of anti-sperm antibodies. Similar conclusions were drawn in 52 male patients by Hellstrom *et al.* (1987).

Soffer *et al.* (1990) cultured chlamydia more frequently from the urethras of normozoospermic rather than oligoasthenoteratozoospermic patients in a group of 175 infertile men. They did, however, demonstrate a greater frequency of anti-sperm antibodies in infected men. On both epidemiological and serological grounds Ruijs *et al.* (1990) concluded from their study of 184 infertile male partners that 'chlamydial infection probably does not contribute significantly to male infertility'.

Neither Torode *et al.* (1987) nor Forsey and Hull (1989) could demonstrate evidence of an increased incidence of antichlamydial antibodies in the serum of women with unexplained infertility. Although Rowland *et al.* (1985) found that the success of IVF was 50 per cent less in women who were sero-positive for chlamydia, Torode *et al.* (1987) failed to confirm these observations.

With respect to the fallopian tube, chlamydia were identified in tissue-cultured specimens obtained from the tubal mucosa in 8 of 34 patients (Maranna *et al.* 1990). Three of these eight had no apparent cause for their infertility. While this study suggests an avenue of further research, its conclusions do not imply that *C. trachomatis* in non-occluded tubes causes infertility. Moreover, the association with tubal pathology could be coincidental, as tubal abnormalities among 184 female partners were correlated with both immunological evidence of chlamydial infection and with the lifetime number of sexual partners (Ruijs *et al.* 1991).

CONCLUSIONS

Undoubtedly, infection of the female with *C. trachomatis* sufficient to cause tubal damage causes infertility. There may be an association between the presence of *U. urealyticum* and *M. hominis* and the formation of anti-sperm antibodies. But, on the basis of the currently available data, it is difficult to support the contention that identification of one of the three micro-organisms discussed in this chapter furnishes an explanation of a couple's infertility.

Definition with respect to infective agents

The identification of the Mycoplasmas, U. urealyticum, *or* C. trachomatis *from either partner does not furnish an explanation for the couple's infertility.*

---

10   Uterine factors

Anatomical distortions of the uterus caused by congenital malformations, fibromyomata, polyps, adhesions, and prenatal exposure to
diethylstilboestrol may be detected by hysterosalpingography, ultrasonography, or hysteroscopy. Occasionally, an overlooked intrauterine contraceptive device may be identified. It is the purpose of this
chapter to describe the means of detection of such lesions, their
prevalence, and whether or not detection of such conditions can be
interpreted as an explanation for infertility.

HISTORY

Disturbances of the menstrual pattern and repeated abortion are
clues suggestive of the presence of uterine lesions. An increased
duration and amount of bleeding associated with a regular menstrual
interval may be reported by women who harbour a uterine malformation. This pattern will usually have been apparent since puberty.
The bleeding associated with fibromyomata occurs later in life, and
worsens as the tumour increases in size. Submucous myomata and
mucus polyps are frequently asymptomatic, but may cause inter-
menstrual spotting.

Intrauterine adhesions may be asymptomatic (Taylor *et al.* 1981)
or, depending on their severity or position in the uterus, cause
amenorrhoea (Asherman 1948). As an aside, the eponymous Asherman's Syndrome was originally described by Fritsch (1894). Hypomenorrhoea may also occur (Sugimoto 1978). Adhesions do not arise
de novo, but rather usually follow some intrauterine event, the most
common of which is postabortal sharp curettage. In cases of amenorrhoea, if intrauterine adhesions are suspected of being causative, the

history is frequently one of the typical menstrual molimina occurring on a regular basis, unaccompanied by menstruation. Confirmation that ovulation is occurring and failure to experience withdrawal bleeding after sequential administration of oestrogen and progesterone confirm the diagnosis. Primary amenorrhoea may suggest congenital absence of the uterus or cervix. Uterine causes of amenorrhoea are reasons for infertility.

A history of maternal ingestion of diethylstilboestrol should arouse suspicion that a T-shaped uterine deformity may exist. Uterine malformations, fibromyomata, adhesions, and the T-shaped uterus may all be identified in women complaining of habitual abortion, although whether adhesions are a cause or an effect remains unclear (Shaffer 1986). All of these lesions may occur in otherwise asymptomatic infertile women.

PHYSICAL EXAMINATION

In the case of uterine malformations or fibromyomata, physical examination may reveal a large, firm, irregularly-shaped uterus. Congenital absence of the uterus can be detected; but, in most cases of infertility, no abnormalities of the uterus will be found by routine pelvic examination.

INVESTIGATIONS

Ultrasonography has been used indiscriminately to 'assess the pelvis', but uterine lesions may be detected from time to time. This technique has yet to be shown to be equivalent to hysterosalpingography as a method of screening for uterine lesions (McArdle and Berezin 1980). Hysteroscopy is to the final diagnosis of uterine lesions as laparoscopy is to the final diagnosis of tubal lesions. Hysteroscopy was the first gynaecological endoscopic procedure to be performed, and was reported by Panteleoni in 1869 (Silander 1963). While simple diagnostic hysteroscopy can be carried out without anaesthesia as an office procedure (Salat-Baroux *et al.* 1984), a logical case can be made for performing hysteroscopy for the investigation of the infertile patient at the time of laparoscopy (Sciarra and Valle 1977; Taylor and Gomel 1986).

If the Hamou (1981) instrument is used, prior cervical dilatation is not required. The distension medium used is carbon dioxide (CO_2). The pressure of the CO_2 is sufficient to dilate the cervix and permit easy passage of the instrument. Usually, views within the uterine cavity are remarkably clear. It is a low-risk procedure if performed correctly. Failure to complete the hysteroscopy occurs in about 4 per cent of cases (Hamou and Taylor 1982). Uterine perforation can occur. Lindemann (1979) reported 6 such events in 5200 cases. If concurrent laparoscopy is being performed, the damage can be assessed immediately, and is almost invariably of little consequence. Infection is rare, occurring seven times in 1000 examinations (Salat-Baroux *et al.* 1984), or not at all among 1500 cases (Lindemann 1979).

PREVALENCE AND SIGNIFICANCE OF UTERINE LESIONS

The frequency of intrauterine lesions detected by hysterosalpingo-graphy and hysteroscopy is shown in Table 10.1. The frequency of congenital malformations is essentially the same regardless of the technique used. As these studies represent selected populations, the prevalence of such lesions (about 4 per cent) is considerably higher than the 1:700 that may be expected in the general population (Glass and Goldbus 1978). Submucous leiomyomata were observed with approximately the same frequency by both methods.

Why should adhesions and polyps appear to occur with eight to ten times the frequency in hysteroscopic examinations that they do in hysterosalpingographic examinations? This may represent an arte-fact produced by the procedure. When a change was made from classic panoramic hysteroscopy to hysteroscopy using the Hamou instrument, the observed prevalence of polyps fell from 12 per cent to 3 per cent, and of adhesions from 22 per cent to 1 per cent (Taylor *et al.* 1987). Both these latter figures correspond closely to the frequency as detected by hysterosalpingography. It was postulated that the cervical dilatation necessary for the performance of panoramic hysteroscopy may have dislodged strips of endometrium, which

Table 10.1 *Frequency of uterine lesions among infertile female partners*

Type of investigation	Adhesions (per cent)	Polyps (per cent)	Fibroids (per cent)	Congenital anomaly (per cent)	*n*	Authors
Hysterosalpingogram	3.0	2.2	3.5	4.8	231	Rice *et al.* 1986
	0.6	0.4	1.6	2.8	505	SanFillippo *et al.* 1978
	0.8	0.4	0	1.2	254	Taylor 1985
Weighted mean	**1.2**	**0.8**	**1.6**	**2.8**		
Hysteroscopy	3.3	16.7	2.4	2.9	210	Gallinat 1984
	11.4	21.0	6.6	5.4	167	Lindemann 1979
	4.7	3.8	2.5	3.8	236	Lubke and Hindenburg 1984
	21.1	11.8	1.6	1.2	837	Taylor 1985
	3.2	0.7	0.4	2.9	278	Taylor *et al.* 1987
	19.7	23.9	7.7	6.3	142	Valle 1980
Weighted mean	**13.4**	**11.4**	**2.5**	**2.7**		

Table 10.2 *Correlation between hysterosalpingogram and hysteroscopy results in the detection of intrauterine lesions*

Number in study	Intrauterine lesions per cent (95 per cent CI)		Kappa value	Sensitivity (per cent)	Specificity (per cent)	Authors
	Normal HSG	Abnormal HSG				
400	1 (0,2)	87 (82,92)	0.86	99	88	Fayez *et al.* 1987
91	31 (8,54)	81 (72,90)	0.41	92	44	Labastida *et al.* 1988
47	30 (10,50)	44 (25,63)	0.14	67	48	Ragni *et al.* 1984
77	2 (0,6)	69 (46,92)	0.74	92	92	Snowden *et al.* 1984
Weighted means			**0.72**	95	79	

were misinterpreted as being intrauterine lesions. Use of the smaller Hamou instrument does not require prior cervical dilatation.

A comparison of the results reported using hysteroscopy and hysterosalpingography in the same patients is shown in Table 10.2. In the largest study, the sensitivity of the hysterosalpingogram was 99 per cent; and the typical sensitivity in these 4 studies was 95 per cent. Reflecting as it does a very low rate of false negatives, this degree of sensitivity would suggest that a normal hysterosalpingogram is very probably accurate with respect to the uterine cavity.

In order to evaluate the usefulness of HSG as a screening test in practice, these diagnostic properties can be applied following the procedures used in Table 5.4. The typical prevalence of intrauterine pathology in these studies with selected patients was 45 per cent. The prevalence is less than 10 per cent in studies based on the use of the microhysteroscope (Taylor *et al.* 1987).

The typical sensitivity and specificity in the published data were 95 and 79 per cent, respectively, and these can be applied to a hypothetical group of 1000 patients, 10 per cent of whom have intrauterine pathology as determined by hysteroscopy (Table 10.3). The calculations indicate that, in the average practice, a normal HSG will be corrected by hysteroscopy in only 1 per cent of cases,

Table 10.3 *Predictive value of HSG in an infertility practice with prevalence of intrauterine lesions equal to 10 per cent*

	Hysteroscopy results		Total
	Lesion	No lesion	
HSG results:			
Lesion present	95[a]	189[b]	284[(a+b)]
No lesion	5[c]	711[d]	716[(c+d)]
Total	100	900	1000

Calculations: [a] 95 per cent (sensitivity) × 100; [c] = 100 − 5;
[d] 79 per cent (specificity) × 900; [b] = 900 − 711;
PPV, 95/284 = 33 per cent (67 per cent of abnormal HSG results will be proved wrong at hysteroscopy);
NPV, 711/716 = 99 per cent (99 per cent of normal HSG results will be proved right at hysteroscopy).

and thus provides about 99 per cent confidence that hysteroscopy is not needed; and such a normal test result would occur in 72 per cent of patients. In the remaining 28 per cent of patients, the abnormal test result would be proved wrong in 67 per cent of hysteroscopies; but, for the majority of patients, the operative procedure would have been avoided or delayed.

Thus hysterosalpingography is a reliable screening investigation for the infertile woman, in whom hysteroscopy need only be used if the hysterosalpingogram apparently reveals a lesion.

Some women are at high risk of harbouring an intrauterine lesion, particularly those with a history of habitual abortion, repeated curettage, or significant alteration of menstrual flow. In these women and those over 35 years of age hysteroscopy may be performed as the primary procedure. This is usually carried out at the same time as the diagnostic laparoscopy.

SUMMARY

Can the detection of an intrauterine lesion be the explanation for a couple's infertility? Congenital malformations have been implicated as a cause of habitual abortion. The rates of abortion have been reported as: bicornuate uterus, 34 per cent; septate uterus, 22 per cent; and unicornuate uterus, 35 per cent (Glass and Goldbus 1978). There is no evidence that such malformations cause infertility. The abortion rate in women with fibromyomata may be as high as 41 per cent, but there is no evidence that fibromyomata cause infertility (Buttram and Reiter 1981). Mucous polyps are observed with the same frequency in women complaining of infertility and those who request reversal sterilization, who are at least of previously proven fertility (Taylor *et al.* 1987). It is difficult to see how polyps might be implicated as causal.

Those adhesions of sufficient severity to cause amenorrhoea or severe hypomenorrhoea probably are causal. Such severe adhesions are fortunately uncommon. Those occurring in eumenorrhoeic women may simply be incidental findings (Taylor *et al.* 1987), nor does maternal ingestion of diethylstilboestrol seem to cause infertility.

Nevertheless, given that congenital malformations, myomata,

and maternal DES ingestion may cause abortion, these lesions should be sought actively and, when necessary, treated. It does not profit the infertile couple to achieve a greatly desired pregnancy only to lose it by a preventable abortion.

Definition

A diagnosis of unexplained infertility is made, with respect to uterine factors, when the presence of severe intrauterine adhesions or congenital absence of the uterus or cervix has been excluded. Other uterine lesions, which may cause habitual abortion, cannot be implicated as causative.

---

11 A final working clinical definition of unexplained infertility and the investigations necessary to establish the diagnosis

Southam (1960) described unexplained infertility as being a 'misfortune due to the laws of chance, or a limitation in our knowledge'. As has been demonstrated in the preceding chapters, when the modern diagnostic assessment is correlated with infertility, it must be apparent that there remains '. . . a limitation in our knowledge'.

This limitation reflects both the inadequacies and lack of scope of the currently available test procedures. Despite these constraints, patients expect a rational diagnostic approach and an explanation of their infertility. It is the purpose of this chapter to define unexplained infertility and the investigation necessary to establish this diagnosis, within the context of the earlier general definition (Chapter 2), which stated: 'unexplained infertility can be said to exist when all tests of the reproductive processes, which are reliable in identifying conditions which can be shown to impair fertility, are normal'.

DEFINITION

Because of the shortcomings of the diagnostic evaluation, it is not possible to be sure of identifying all possible causes of infertility in any given couple. The best that can be hoped for is to detect one or more lesions which are known to be causative. Even if such lesions are detected, there are no guarantees that other factors which are also contributing to the infertility are not operative.

Nevertheless, if such obvious lesions are detected, the diagnosis of unexplained infertility is excluded. It makes sense to conduct the investigation of the infertile couple in a way which will uncover such lesions.

During the course of this investigation, test results in some couples will lie outside the normal range, without in themselves adequately explaining the infertility. And yet, in the face of such findings, a diagnosis of unexplained infertility cannot honestly be made.

At the conclusion of the investigation of any group of couples, a final subgroup will remain; those in whom neither definite causes nor abnormal test results have been identified. This subgroup of couples have unexplained infertility.

For practical clinical purposes, it is necessary to move from the rigid categorizing of couples as either explained or unexplained, and to consider a more realistic classification of infertility as:

(1) probably explained—a causative lesion has been detected;

(2) possibly explained—test result(s) lie outside the normal range; or

(3) unexplained—no abnormal test results have been identified.

INVESTIGATIONS

The investigation should be arranged in such a way as to identify those conditions which are probable causes of infertility. As the search for these probable causes progresses, some possible causes may also be identified. Before beginning it is helpful to take note of the probable and possible causes of infertility, as listed in Table 11.1.

An investigation which would ensure the identification of the conditions listed in Table 11.1 requires history-taking, examination of the female, and specific test procedures. It cannot be stressed too strongly that, as infertility affects couples, the physician intending to care for such patients must insist that the couple will be interviewed together at the first visit, and that subsequent management will be designed to meet the needs of both partners.

Table 11.1 *Probable and possible causes of infertility*

Mechanism	Probable cause	Possible cause
Ovulation	Anovulation	Irregular cycles
Spermatogenesis and sperm transport in the male	Azoospermia Aspermia Sperm count $< 5 \times 10^6$/ml Progressive motility < 20 per cent Normal morphology < 20 per cent	Sperm count 5 to 20×10^6/ml Progressive motility 20 to 50 per cent Normal morphology 20 to 50 per cent
Sperm and oocyte transport in the female	Tubal occlusion Endometriosis Stages III and IV	Tubal adhesions (tubes patent) Endometriosis Stages I and II
Uterine factors	Congenital absence Dense uterine adhesions	——
Sexual function	Apareunia	Coital dysfunction

History-taking

The importance of age (particularly of the female partner), duration of infertility, and previous reproductive history have been described. This information must be recorded.

The menstrual pattern of the female partner should be determined. If the following information is obtained some inferences can be drawn.

(a) Regular cycles of 25–35 day intervals—95 per cent probability that ovulation is occurring

(b) Amenorrhoea—anovulation, destruction of the endometrium, absence of the uterus, or obstruction to menstrual flow

(c) Cycle length greater than 35 days—possible anovulation

(d) Heavy regular flow—of early onset, possible uterine malformation—of late onset, possible uterine fibromyomata or endometriosis

(e) Abnormalities in the pattern of flow which are of recent onset—possible endometriosis or chronic pelvic inflammatory changes

(f) Pre-menstrual molimina (including breast tenderness, bloating, and mood changes)—suggestive of ovulatory cycles

The patient may complain of pelvic pain. While primary dysmenorrhoea and *Mittelschmerz* are suggestive of ovulatory cycles, secondary dysmenorrhoea, chronic acyclic pelvic pain, and deep dyspareunia may be associated with chronic pelvic inflammatory changes or endometriosis. It must be remembered that these conditions can also be asymptomatic.

Attention should be paid to any previous surgical history, particularly of appendectomy, gynaecological procedures, pelvic operations, or repeated dilatation and curettage. The first three may be associated with chronic pelvic adhesive disease, the last with intrauterine adhesions. The general medical history is rarely of help in determining the cause of infertility unless anovulation is present. A history of sexually transmitted disease is significant. The rubella status should be determined, and if unknown it should be tested (Leader *et al.* 1985). Women who are not immune should be immunized.

Previous contraceptive use should be noted. Use of the oral contraceptive does not cause infertility, but may slightly prolong the discontinuation to conception interval (Vessey *et al*. 1976). Use of the intrauterine contraceptive device, if associated with complications, may have resulted in pelvic inflammatory changes. Occasionally, a woman may think such a device has been removed when in fact it remains *in situ*. Removal can have remarkably curative powers. Social habits, including alcohol, cigarette, and street-drug consumption should be noted. Cigarette smoking appears to reduce fecundability, an effect that may worsen as the cigarette consumption increases (Weinberg *et al*. 1989). The family history may reveal the presence of heritable disease. While such disorders may not directly affect fertility, they may have implications should pregnancy occur. A history of endometriosis in a first-degree relative is noteworthy.

Demographic information (age, occupation) and the previous reproductive history of the male partner must be noted. This history should focus on possible reasons for impairment of spermatogenesis. Developmental problems include intrauterine exposure to diethylstilboestrol, undescended testes, and delayed onset of puberty. Events occurring during adult life, such as post-pubertal mumps infection, alcohol, tobacco, and other substance-abuse, symptoms of any systemic endocrinopathy or severe systemic disease, anosmia, and exposure to radiation, chemicals, toxins, and excessive heat, should be sought.

Impaired sperm transport may be suspected if there is a history of inguinal herniorrhaphy (particularly in childhood), sexually transmitted diseases, diabetes mellitus, neurological disorders, or surgery to the bladder neck.

The sexual history should be obtained. The frequency of coitus, timing of coitus, and any coital difficulties should be noted, including impotence or premature ejaculation. Severe coital difficulties are a cause of infertility. Deep dyspareunia indicates the possible presence of endometriosis or chronic pelvic inflammatory changes.

PHYSICAL EXAMINATION

It is not necessary to examine the male partner unless subsequent evaluation of the ejaculate demonstrates azoospermia (Dunphy *et al.* 1989*a*).

The female partner should be examined. While the examination should be thorough, it is not necessary to describe here the routine physical examination. Patients in whom the menstrual history is suggestive of anovulation should be evaluated specifically for any general stigmata of endocrinopathy or chromosomal or systemic disorders. In all patients, particular attention should be paid to the abdominal and pelvic examinations. The presence of abdominal scars should be noted. Appendectomy and pelvic surgery may have lead to periadnexal adhesion formation. Any areas of tenderness should be noted.

The pelvic examination should evaluate the position, size, shape, consistency, and mobility of the uterus. Mobile retroversion is not a cause of infertility. Fixed retroversion could be an indication that chronic pelvic inflammatory changes or endometriosis are present. Firm, irregular enlargement of the uterus suggests the presence of leiomyomata. Palpation of the adnexa will reveal any major degree of ovarian enlargement. Tenderness or nodularity of the pelvic peritoneum raises the index of suspicion that endometriosis might be present, as does such a finding at the time of the recto-vaginal examination.

INVESTIGATION

While of no value in the diagnosis of possible cause, it is at this point, when the history and physical examination have been completed, that the process of decision-making with the couple begins. It is now incumbent upon the physician to determine as clearly as possible their needs. On the basis of the history, physical findings, and perceived needs, the investigation to be performed should be decided upon, and the probable course of action should be described. The feelings of helplessness experienced by most infertile couples can be greatly ameliorated if they can understand what is to be done and why. Investigations should be performed as rapidly, accurately, and inexpensively as possible.

Laboratory test which would be indicated by incidental findings of the history and physical examination may be necessary. The specific investigation for infertility should be directed initially towards the detection of abnormalities of ovulation in the female and spermatogenesis and sperm transport in the male.

During the first consultation, the likelihood that ovulation is occurring can be ascertained initially from the menstrual history. Cycle length of 25–35 days is excellent presumptive evidence. A single mid-luteal progesterone value equal to or exceeding 16 nmol/l is all that is required as confirmation. For a small number of patients, the use of the basal body temperature graph may be more convenient than blood sampling. Patients with a cycle length greater than 35 days will require weekly samples to be drawn for progesterone measurement during the probable time of the luteal phase. Sampling in such patients should commence on day 21 and be performed at 7-day intervals. If anovulation is detected, a probable cause of the infertility has been identified. If ovulation is occurring, measurement of thyroid and gonadotrophic hormones and prolactin is wasteful and adds no information of value (Conway *et al*. 1985).

At the same time, two semen analyses should be performed, and three broad categories of results can be anticipated.

If the man has azoospermia or results falling below either 5 million sperm/ml, and/or 20 per cent progressive motility, and/or 20 per cent normal forms, a probable cause for the infertility has been identified. The second category includes those in whom one or more of the classical parameters, while exceeding the minimum cutpoints, may fall below the currently accepted norms (WHO 1987). In these cases, a possible cause of infertility has been identified. Or, finally, all the classic parameters may meet or exceed the currently accepted norms.

At this point, these couples in whom abnormalities of ovulation or spermatogenesis or sperm transport in the male have been detected are by definition excluded from the category of unexplained infertility. They will, of course require further investigation and management, both of which are beyond the scope of this book.

In the third category there are no abnormal findings at this point, and attention must now be focused upon evaluating sperm and oocyte transport in the female and the presence or absence of endometriosis.

Sperm and oocyte transport in the upper genital tract of the female are initially evaluated by hysterosalpingography (HSG). For those patients in whom historical or physical findings are suggestive of an intrapelvic or intrauterine lesion, and in women of 35 years or older or in whom the infertility is of long duration, hysterosalpingography should be replaced by immediate recourse to laparoscopy combined with hysteroscopy.

The HSG will either be normal or abnormal. If it is abnormal, immediate laparoscopy and, if a uterine lesion is suspected, hysteroscopy should be performed. If the HSG is normal, laparoscopic evaluation should be delayed for six months. During this time, some couples will achieve a spontaneous pregnancy. Until the laparoscopy has been performed, and shown to be normal, a diagnosis of unexplained infertility cannot be made.

Once the laparoscopy and, where necessary, the hysteroscopy have been completed, four broad categories of patients will be identified. Some women will have tubal occlusion, or severe periadnexal disease, or Stage III or Stage IV endometriosis will have been identified. In these couples, the infertility is probably explained. The second category of women will have periadnexal adhesions or Stage I or Stage II endometriosis. Such couples have possibly explained infertility. A third group will have lesions of the uterine cavity that do *not* cause infertility, but may require management as prophylaxis against abortion. Only in the fourth category, where no lesions are identified, can the couple be considered to have unexplained infertility.

Thus a simple investigative protocol will allow identification of all the probable causes of infertility, all of which will require further investigation and management.

It will further identify a group of couples with possibly explained infertility who also may require further investigation and management. The further treatment of couples with probable and possible causes of infertility is beyond the scope of this book.

Because in the remainder of couples ovulation has been confirmed, the seminal analysis parameters are normal, and laparoscopy has failed to reveal any abnormality, a diagnosis of unexplained infertility can now be made.

Should further investigations be performed? Discouraging though it may be to physicians and frustrating as it is to the patients, it would appear from the data presented in the preceding chapters that, while many investigations are of interest and may, in the future, add further insight, none at present seems to alter the outcome for any individual couple.

Search for the luteal phase defect by histological or hormonal evaluation has not been productive. The postcoital test 'lacks validity as a test for infertility' (Griffith and Grimes 1990). Computerized measurements of sperm-movement characteristics have yet to produce a simple but discriminating variable which independently relates to fertility. Nor does the use of the zona-free hamster ova test significantly improve the prediction of fertility. *In vitro* fertilization may be a useful further diagnostic assessment, but it is not practical for this purpose alone. No clear correlations have been demonstrated between anti-sperm antibody presence and fertility. And the finding of *Mycoplasma* or *Chlamydia* does not identify a cause for infertility.

It would seem, therefore, that in clinical practice today the diagnosis of unexplained infertility can be made on the basis of the clinical findings and investigations described in this chapter.

12 The prognosis for couples with unexplained infertility

INTRODUCTION

The definition of unexplained infertility that we have supplied may not be unanimously accepted, but clinical decision-making must go on, and such decisions should be based, as was our definition, on the published evidence. Before any treatment of unexplained infertility is chosen, it must be demonstrably superior to the no-treatment option. The prognosis for untreated unexplained infertility can be very good or can be discouraging, depending on the characteristics of each individual couple. This chapter will evaluate the published experience to describe the prognosis for untreated unexplained infertility, and those factors in the individual couple which may influence the prognosis.

The chapter begins by describing the methods which should be applied in follow-up studies in order for such studies to serve as the basis from which to derive accurate prognostic information. A discussion of pregnancy rates during follow-up and the clinical and other factors that affect pregnancy rates follows. The chapter concludes by illustrating how this information can be used to formulate a prognosis for untreated unexplained infertility that is specific to the individual couple.

METHODS FOR THE STUDY OF FOLLOW-UP OBSERVATIONS

The literature to date is variable in its use of definitions and diagnostic protocols; but in virtually every study the inclusion criteria have specified evaluation of ovulation, semen analysis, and laparoscopy.

There was less consistency with respect to the use of postcoital tests, endometrial biopsies, microbiological tests, hysteroscopy, and anti-sperm antibody tests before a diagnosis of unexplained infertility could be made (Table 12.1). The majority of published clinical reports fall under the heading of descriptive studies, consisting of case series which are usually non-comparative in nature. The usefulness of such studies lies in their ability to provide information about the outcome of a clinical disorder, such as infertility. They are useless for evaluating treatment efficacy, but may provide important information about the side-effects and complications of treatment that could occur during follow-up. The important issues in the design of such studies deal with the assembly or recruitment of subjects, the methods of follow-up, the outcome assessment, and the analysis, which, in the case of a chronic disorder such as infertility, is usually some form of survival analysis.

Assembly of cases

Case series may be assembled retrospectively or prospectively, but any such studies will have more value when the inclusion and exclusion criteria are established prior to the assembly of cases, and the criteria should, of course, be meticulously followed. The diagnostic protocol should rule out similar but ineligible conditions, and the information available at the starting-point should include all relevant demographic and clinical detail. Exclusion criteria should be explicit. In the case of infertility, for example, a previous sterilization of either partner or less than 12 months without contraception would constitute exclusion criteria. Compromises may be necessary. In a case series, a balance must be struck between a small, extremely homogeneous group for the study of a specific element, and a larger, more varied group of subjects, which would be more representative of clinical practice in general. Thus the use of extensive and strict inclusion and exclusion criteria may mean that the results of a given study will be more credible with respect to a particular factor; but the exclusion of many subjects who are made ineligible by these restrictions may also mean that the remainder will be less typical of infertile subjects in general.

Table 12.1 *Diagnostic protocols in reports on the prognosis for untreated couples with unexplained infertility*

Authors	Number of patients	Semen analysis	Serum progesterone or endometrial biopsy	Hysterosalpingogram	Laparoscopy	Postcoital test	Antisperm antibody
Aitken et al. 1984	68	✓	✓	.	✓	.	.
Barnea et al. 1985	58	✓	.	✓	.	✓	.
Check et al. 1989	50	✓	✓	.	✓	✓	.
Collins 1989	340	✓	✓	✓	✓	.	.
Daly 1989	47	✓	✓	✓	✓	✓	.
Dor et al. 1977	117	✓	✓	✓	.	✓	.
Fisch et al. 1989	36	✓	✓	✓	✓	.	.
Glazener et al. 1987c	176	✓	✓	.	✓	✓	.
Hull et al. 1985	196	✓	✓	.	✓	✓	.
Iffland et al. 1989	17	✓	✓	.	✓	✓	✓
Kliger 1984	127	✓	✓	✓	✓	✓	.
Lenton et al. 1977	96	✓	✓	✓	✓	✓	.
Rousseau et al. 1983	47	✓	✓	✓	✓	.	.
Sorensen 1980	36	✓	✓	✓	.	✓	.
Southam 1960	312	✓	✓	✓	.	.	.
Templeton and Penney 1982	124	✓	✓	.	✓	.	.
Trimbos-Kemper et al. 1984	89	✓	✓	✓	✓	✓	.
Van Dijk et al. 1979	19	✓	✓	✓	✓	✓	.
Welner et al. 1988	48	✓	✓	✓	✓	✓	.
Wright et al. 1979	23	✓	✓	.	✓	✓	.
	2026	20	19	13	16	13	1

Follow-up

Careful follow-up always begins with a definite starting-point. For the study of infertility, two choices are available; the date at which conception attempts started, or the date when observations in the relevant clinical care setting began. In the case of treatment studies, the start date may coincide with the first date of treatment. Because detailed recordings are only possible during the period of direct observation, the majority of studies choose as a starting-point the date of registration or first visit to the clinical care setting. Widely spaced intervals of contact tend to lead to loss of follow-up, while over-frequent follow-up visits can lead to non-compliance. Because the incidence of interurban mobility in the reproductive age-group is high, follow-up at three-month intervals is often indicated to ensure that contact is maintained with the maximum number of subjects.

Outcome assessment

A revealing measure of the quality of any clinical follow-up study is the completeness of the outcome assessment. All the clinically relevant elements should be reported in sufficient detail to indicate what happened to each subject. In studies of infertility, the primary outcome of interest is pregnancy, which may or may not occur. For subjects who conceive, other outcomes are also important, and these include the rates of live births, perinatal deaths, abortions, and ectopic pregnancies. For those who do not conceive, other events that are related to the purpose of the study include loss to follow-up, adoption, and resolution of the need to pursue further investigation or treatment.

Where the duration of follow-up is reasonably short, a simple statement of the proportion of subjects who experience each relevant outcome provides the most important clinical information. Thus, in a given study, the pregnancy rate after six months might be 10 per cent. While this figure is accurate for the individual study population, it may or may not truly represent the outcome to be expected in other similar groups. The 95 per cent confidence interval of that 10 per cent estimate describes the range of possibilities that might be found in other similar groups.

Often the follow-up is longer than an arbitrary six months, and it is important to understand the distribution of the outcomes of interest throughout the time of observation. They can more accurately be described by means of survival analysis.

Survival analysis is a class of statistical procedures which is useful for estimating the frequency with which an event will occur during a period of time. In studies of infertility, the simplest and most important end-point is conception or no conception, and this clear-cut dichotomous outcome is most appropriately analysed with the use of life tables, the most elementary type of survival analysis. The life table can also be used to evaluate the effect of a limited number of factors which might affect whether or not conception occurred (Mantel 1966). If a larger number of potentially influential factors needs to be assessed simultaneously, multivariate forms of survival analysis can be used. In clinical studies of infertility, the proportional hazards model is most frequently used (Cox 1972).

One of the most valuable pieces of information that can be generated from clinical studies is the relative risk. Simply stated, this term describes the probability that an event will occur more or less frequently in one group when compared with another. If the relative risk for conception is 1.6, for example, in women of less than 30 years of age, compared with women of 30 years or older, then the younger woman is 1.6 times more likely to conceive. With multivariate analysis, the relative risk can be calculated taking into account additional variables which might influence the prognosis. The expression of the relative risk, with its confidence limits, can then be directly applied in clinical decision-making.

PREGNANCY RATES DURING FOLLOW-UP OF UNTREATED UNEXPLAINED INFERTILITY

Twenty reports or case series provide information about the prognosis for pregnancy among untreated couples with unexplained infertility (Table 12.2). In seven of these, the data represent the outcome for the untreated groups in comparative studies (Check *et al.* 1989; Daly 1989; Fisch *et al.* 1989; Iffland *et al.* 1989; Van Dijk *et al.* 1979; Welner *et al.* 1988; Wright *et al.* 1979). The remainder

Table 12.2 *Reports on the prognosis for pregnancy among untreated couples with unexplained infertility*

Authors	Number of patients	Mean duration of infertility (m)	Mean female age (y)	Primary infertility (per cent)	Maximum months of FU*	Pregnancy per cent (95 per cent CI)
Aitken et al. 1984	68	62	.	.	30	37 (25,48)
Barnea et al. 1985	58	39	29	.	60	79 (69,90)
Check et al. 1989	50	.	.	.	8	16 (6,26)
Collins 1989	340	39	30	75	48	34 (29,39)
Daly 1989	47	44	31	72	17	43 (57,28)
Dor et al. 1977	117	.	.	50	.	75 (67,83)
Fisch et al. 1989	36	51	30	0	4	0
Glazener et al. 1987c	176	20	28	.	18	.
Hull et al. 1985	196	29	28	60	24	.
Iffland et al. 1989	17	59	31	100	5	6 (0,17)
Kliger 1984	127	38	27	39	84	69 (60,77)
Lenton et al. 1977	96	.	26	89	60	43 (33,53)
Rousseau et al. 1983	47	50	28	83	84	57 (43,72)
Sorenson 1980	36	40	27	56	100	53 (37,69)
Southam 1960	312	.	.	.	.	19 (15,24)
Templeton and Penney 1982	124	35	27	73	.	49 (40, 58)
Trimbos-Kemper et al. 1984	89	54	29	82	60	43 (34,54)
Van Dijk et al. 1979	19	66	30	84	6	5 (0,15)
Welner et al. 1988	48	78	31	90	140	4 (0,10)
Wright et al. 1979	23	58	30	100	6	22 (5,39)
Weighted means	(2026 couples)	40	29	70	46	33

* FU: follow-up

are case series of untreated subjects. The main clinical findings in these studies are summarized in Table 12.2. The studies included observations on from 17 to 340 untreated couples; the maximum number of months of follow-up ranged from 4 months to 140 months, and the weighted mean was 43 months. Observed pregnancy rates ranged from 0 to 79 per cent. The weighted mean was 31 per cent. These percentages represent simple statements of the proportion of subjects who conceived.

The lowest pregnancy rate was seen in a study of 4 months' duration, and the highest in a study of 60 months' duration. Clearly a factor influencing the published pregnancy rate is the duration of follow-up. Other factors which might have accounted for differences in the reported pregnancy rates include sample size, mean duration of infertility, mean age of female partners, and the percentage of patients with primary infertility in each study group. When multiple regression analysis was performed, the mean duration of infertility was found to account for 73 per cent of the variability in the reported pregnancy rates. The number of months of follow-up contributed a further 13 per cent.

Two large studies made use of life-table analysis to refine the estimate of fertility further. Among 196 couples with unexplained infertility observed in a Bristol clinic the mean duration of infertility was 29 months. The cumulative pregnancy rate was 72 per cent after 24 months (Hull *et al*. 1985). The mean duration of infertility was 39 months among 340 couples followed in Canadian infertility clinics for up to 42 months (mean length of follow-up was 22 months). The simple pregnancy rate was 34 per cent, and the cumulative pregnancy rate at 36 months after registration was 46 per cent ± 4 per cent (Collins 1989*b*). It should be recognized that, when the life-table analysis is used, the cumulative pregnancy rates will usually exceed the simple pregnancy rate, because life-table analysis corrects for patients who are lost to follow-up. When simple pregnancy rates are calculated, patients lost to follow-up are regarded as not pregnant; life-table analysis implies that lost subjects have the same experience as those whose outcomes are known.

Reports on infertility treatment frequently express the prognosis in terms of fecundability, or the potential for live birth per cycle. This strict definition is often altered: conceptions may be substituted for live births, and fecundability may be expressed per 100 cycles, or per cent per cycle. When such results are reported for untreated couples, they are derived from months of observation rather than cycles, and should be interpreted as approximate fecundability. A typical rate (2.1 per cent per 100 months) was reported by Murdoch *et al.* (1991) among 73 couples with unexplained infertility (median duration five years) who were observed for 894 months. Table 12.3 illustrates how fecundability declines from 5 to 1 per cent per month as the duration of infertility increases from one to more than five years.

The concept of fecundability does not serve well as a basis for comparison with pregnancy rates per cycle of treatment. Events during long periods of observation are not comparable with the results of a few cycles of therapy, for reasons that will be discussed in Chapter 15. Expressing the prognosis for untreated unexplained infertility in this way, however, brings immediacy to the prognosis and more realism to the expectations of the couple as each month passes.

It is useful to know either the simple or cumulative pregnancy rate in the medium term or the fecundability for the average couple with unexplained infertility. A much more accurate prognosis can be given to the individual couple if it also takes into account other factors in the couple that may affect the average prognosis; these include the duration of infertility, age, pregnancy history, coital frequency, and social class.

Table 12.3 *Approximate fecundability with untreated unexplained infertility**

Duration of infertility (years)	Number of cases	Mean duration of infertility (months)	Secondary infertility (per cent)	Mean female age (years)	Pregnancy rate (per 100 months)
one to two	101	16	30	30.2	5.1
two to three	89	26	24	29.0	2.9
three to four	102	40	25	29.5	2.2
five or more	89	78	21	31.4	1.0
Total	381	160	25	30.0	2.7

* Data from the Canadian Infertility Therapy Evaluation Study (Vutyavanich and Collins 1991)

Factors which affect the pregnancy rate

Duration of infertility

The duration of infertility is defined as the length of time during which the couple have had coitus without the use of contraception. To a certain extent, this is a misnomer, as the definition of infertility is not fulfilled until after the first 12 months without contraception. The conventional interpretation will be used here—that is, the total number of months during which the couple has had intercourse without the use of contraception before their first visit to the reporting clinic.

Ninety per cent of couples in an unevaluated population will be expected to conceive within 12 months (Tietze 1956). Stated differently, half of all never-pregnant patients will conceive within the first five months, half of the remainder within the next five months, and after ten months half of those yet remaining will conceive within the following five months (Keller *et al.* 1984). In couples who have previously conceived, the rate is more rapid, and it is predicted that 50 per cent would be pregnant within 3 months. It might be reasonable to suggest that, among couples with unexplained infertility, those who conceive reasonably soon after the diagnosis has been confirmed represent couples in whom chance or a minor self-correcting abnormality is operative. In those who do not conceive after the passage of a reasonable amount of time, some more major factor is likely to be responsible, and by logical extension, the prognosis would be worse.

The mean duration of infertility for the reports in Table 12.2 ranged from 20 months to 84 months. In individual studies, duration of infertility was a significant prognostic factor (Collins 1989*b*; Hull *et al.* 1975; Kliger 1984; Lenton *et al.* 1977; Rousseau *et al.* 1983; Sorensen 1980). The pregnancy rate appeared to be approximately 2 per cent lower for every month of infertility among a group of untreated couples with a mean 39 months' duration of infertility (Collins 1989*b*). This represents a decrease of more than 10 per cent in the expected pregnancy rate for every additional year of infertility in excess of 39 months.

The age factor

Age of the female partner

Information derived from donor insemination programmes has demonstrated a gradual reduction in fertility related to female age. After the age of 30, the probability of pregnancy declines, and the chance of a woman aged 35 years having a healthy newborn is about half that of a woman aged 25 (Van Noord-Zaadstra *et al.* 1991). Pregnancy rates after 12 cycles of treatment were 74 per cent, 61 per cent, and 54 per cent of women aged less than 31 years, of 31 to 35 years, and older than 35 years respectively (Schwartz and Mayaux 1982).

This figure of 54 per cent in the older patients is strikingly similar to that noted by Hull *et al.* (1985). These authors observed that cumulative conception rates in couples with unexplained infertility were 66 per cent to 79 per cent in the lower age-ranges, but were only 51 per cent where the female partner was 35 years of age or more ($p < 0.01$).

In a report where 44 per cent of the women were aged more than 30 years at the time of registration, pregnancy was more likely among younger women; but the independent influence of the female partner's age was significant only in those couples where the duration of infertility exceeded 3 years (Collins and Rowe 1989). Among couples whose duration of infertility exceeded 3 years, the mean age of the female partners was 26 years when they began to try to conceive, and the cumulative pregnancy rate after 24 months was 28 per cent. The effect of aging, as estimated with the use of proportional hazards analysis, indicated that the chance of conception was reduced by a factor of 0.9, or about 2 per cent, below the observed 28 per cent for every year of the female partner's age beyond the mean of 26 years (Collins and Rowe 1989). While other estimates of the effect of age on the prevalence of infertility and on its prognosis have suggested only a modest impact (Aral and Cates 1983; Menken *et al.* 1986), the relatively unimpeded effects of age among couples with persistent unexplained infertility are measurable, significant, and clinically potent.

Age of the male partner

No study to date has revealed an association between the age of the male partner and the pregnancy rate among couples with unexplained infertility. When the age of the male partner was entered into a proportional hazards analysis, this factor was not a significant predictor ($p = 0.29$) of pregnancy among untreated couples with unexplained infertility (Collins 1989*b*). If there was any effect of the age of the male partner, such an effect would probably be non-specific, and could be related to the age of the female partner. Certainly fecundity in the partners of men under 25 years of age is higher (75 per cent in 6 months) than it is for men 40 years or older (25 per cent in six months) (Seibel 1990). Whether this represents a declining fertilizing capability of the male, concomitant aging of the female partner, or a reduction in the frequency of intercourse, is unclear.

Previous reproductive history

If a couple has previously been able to conceive, then at some time all the necessary prerequisites for the initiation of pregnancy were functioning normally. It would seem reasonable to expect that their prognosis might be better.

Lenton *et al.* (1977) reported that cumulative pregnancy rates after 7 years were 36 and 79 per cent in couples with primary and secondary infertility, respectively. After 9 years of follow-up, Templeton and Penney (1982) also observed lower cumulative pregnancy rates with primary infertility (64 per cent) compared with secondary infertility (79 per cent). A proportional hazards analysis accounting for other predictive variables evaluated the pregnancy rate with secondary infertility among untreated couples with unexplained infertility. The pregnancy rate with secondary infertility, defined as a previous pregnancy in the present relationship, was nearly double the pregnancy rate with primary infertility (Collins 1989).

Coital frequency

Conception rates have been correlated to the frequency of intercourse over a six-month period (MacLeod and Gold 1953). The pregnancy rate was less than 20 per cent with coital frequency less than once per week, rising to approximately 50 per cent with coital frequency 3 or more times weekly. It would appear that, while reduced coital frequency may delay the occurrence of pregnancy, even such a low coital frequency as once weekly is not a direct cause of infertility. When coitus does not occur for psychological or other reasons, it may constitute the principal cause of infertility. Coital failure was found to be the major cause of infertility in only 10 of 551 couples (2 per cent) (Hull *et al*. 1985). Reduced coital frequency was not, however, different in the unexplained group, compared with tubal infertility (Templeton and Penney 1982).

Coital frequency of less than twice per week was a significant independent predictor of a lower pregnancy rate in a proportional hazards analysis of 2106 couples (Vutyavanich and Collins 1991). Among 340 untreated couples with unexplained infertility, infrequent coitus was also associated with a reduced likelihood of pregnancy. The relative risk was 0.8 (95 per cent CI: 0.4, 1.6), adjusted for the duration of infertility, female partner's age, and pregnancy history. In this smaller sample, however, the confidence limits of the estimate include unity, so that the possibility that coital frequency has no effect on the prognosis for unexplained infertility has not been excluded with conventional confidence.

Social class

The possibility exists that the older age of the female partner among couples with unexplained infertility (compared with other infertility diagnosis) may arise from different social-class groupings (Collins and Rowe 1989; Menken *et al*. 1986). There were no differences in social class in a report from Scotland, when unexplained infertility and other infertility diagnoses were compared (Templeton and Penney 1982). In the Canadian data, the occupations of couples were compared with a contemporary 1986 subcensus listing occupations in Canada by sex, age, and region. There were more couples with professional occupations and higher income in the infertile group compared with age-matched employed individuals in Canada. This was due to a significant excess of female health professionals among the infertile couples. In the unexplained group, this excess was further exaggerated, but the difference between infertile couples in general and those with unexplained infertility was not significant.

Higher income was significantly associated with better fertility in the analysis of all diagnostic groups, and the trend was also present within the couples whose infertility was unexplained, though in this smaller group it was not significant (Vutyavanich and Collins 1991). The relative probability of pregnancy in the group with better than average income (over $43 000 in 1986 Canadian dollars) was 1.3 (95 per cent CI: 0.9, 1.9); although the point estimate of the effect of income suggests a 30 per cent better prognosis, the lower 95 per cent confidence limit does not rule out the possibility of a small negative effect.

OTHER OUTCOMES

The outcome of pregnancy for couples with unexplained infertility is similar to the outcome expected in couples conceiving without infertility (Lenton *et al.* 1977; Templeton and Penney 1982). In the CITES data, among the 123 couples (32 per cent) who conceived there were 84 live births and 21 abortions. There were 6 pre-term deliveries, and equal numbers of perinatal deaths and ectopic pregnancies (Table 12.4).

Table 12.4 *Pregnancy and other events among 381 untreated couples with unexplained infertility*

Outcome	Number of couples	Percentage of pregnancies	Percentage of couples
Pregnancy	123		32
Live birth	84	68	22
Abortion	21	17	6
Premature birth	6	5	2
Perinatal death	6	5	2
Ectopic pregnancy	6	5	2
Continuing follow-up	127		33
Lost to follow-up	94		25
Resolved	29		8
Adopted	8		2

Data from the Canadian Infertility Therapy Evaluation Study (Vutyavanich and Collins 1991)

Conception is only one of several possible outcomes for an infertile couple; they may adopt, or they may become lost to follow-up, or they may resolve their concern about infertility. During the CITES observation period 2 per cent of the couples with unexplained infertility adopted, 25 per cent were lost to follow-up, and 7 per cent resolved their concern about infertility. The clinical factors related to these other outcomes have not previously been reported. The results of survival analyses of the CITES data will now be discussed.

None of the 11 couples (2 per cent) who adopted during the period of observation had secondary infertility. Higher family income significantly increased the probability of adoption by 54 per cent for every \$10 000 ($p = 0.005$).

The likelihood of loss to follow-up was not significantly associated with the clinical factors that are related to conception, such as duration of infertility, female age, pregnancy history, coital frequency, family income, or laparoscopy status. Loss to follow-up was 40 per cent lower in the treated group, but the significance was marginal ($p = 0.055$).

With respect to resolution, couples with infrequent intercourse were 1.9 times more likely to resolve than those with more frequent intercourse patterns, but the p value for this term was 0.091.

In order better to understand the outcome for couples with infertility, well-designed studies should take into account these competing end-points, and such studies should include more detailed assessments of the clinical and other characteristics that might contribute to one or more of the outcomes.

SUMMARY OF THE PROGNOSIS FOR PREGNANCY

The effect of time on the prognosis for pregnancy is powerful and clinically important. As each year goes by, patients conceive, and in the denominator of couples remaining there is a shift toward dominance by couples with a poor prognosis. Thus with increasing duration of infertility there is a gradual decline in the pregnancy rate that may be expected for the individual couple.

Two data sources showing this trend are published data for mean

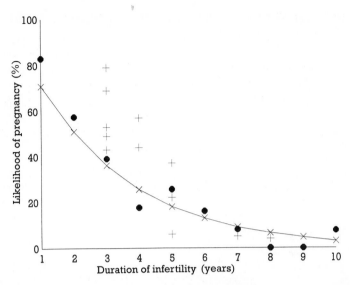

Fig. 12.1 *Duration of infertility and the likelihood of pregnancy among untreated couples with unexplained infertility. Percentage pregnant according to: (1) reported mean duration of infertility (Table 12.2): (+); (2) total waiting-time (duration of infertility at registration plus time under observation after registration) among 381 couples (Collins 1989): (●); (3) total waiting-time among 381 couples, adjusted for other clinical variables: (—×—).*

duration of infertility and pregnancy rate from Table 12.2 and the CITES data for pregnancy rate by total waiting-time (Fig. 12.1). Although the published data seem unreliable in the lower range of mean duration (the intercept would be equivalent to a pregnancy rate of 191 per cent), both sources show similar effects of prolonged duration of infertility on prognosis. The effect of other clinical prognostic factors can be interpreted with the use of the curved regression line obtained from the CITES data, which is seen to fit the unadjusted simple pregnancy rates.

When the duration of infertility is brief, the very good prognosis may be independent of the effect of other factors. After seven or eight years' duration of infertility, the effect of other factors would be quite small, given the very poor prognosis among such couples. With duration of infertility in the middle range, however, the effect of other factors can be superimposed on the prognostic curve shown

Table 12.5 *The effect of clinical characteristics on the probability of pregnancy among 381 couples with unexplained infertility*

Clinical characteristics at the time of registration	Probability of pregnancy (95 per cent CI)	*p* value
Duration of infertility (years)	0.74 (0.64, 0.84)	0.0001
Secondary infertility	2.4 (1.6, 3.7)	0.0001
Female partner's age (years)	0.91 (0.84, 0.97)	0.006
Family income more than $43 000*	1.3 (0.9, 1.9)	0.11
Coitus less than twice per week	0.8 (0.4, 1.4)	0.18
Male partner less than 40 years of age	1.0 (0.5, 2.0)	0.98
(Duration of infertility less than 3 years)†	2.3 (1.4, 3.6)	0.0004
(Female partner's less than 30 years)	1.6 (1.1, 2.4)	0.008

* 1986 Canadian dollars.

† The duration and female age variables were converted to two groups (above and below average), and evaluated in a separate analysis including pregnancy history, income, coital history, and male age. Also included in each Cox analysis was the variable for time to laparoscopy.

in Fig. 12.1. Older female age would place the couple below the curve; the history of a pregnancy in the partnership would place the couple above the curve; and decreased coital frequency would probably diminish the prognosis, although that effect has not been demonstrated with conventional clinical significance.

Values for such approximate adjustments can be based on survival data as summarized in Table 12.5. The pregnancy rate is reduced by 26 per cent for every additional year of infertility, as is also shown in Fig. 12.1, where pregnancy rate declines approximately 26 per cent, from 51 per cent after two years' to 39 per cent after three years' duration of infertility. In some cases the effect of duration can be stated more simply; if the duration is less than three years the prognosis is 2.3 times better than average. With secondary infertility, the prognosis is 2.4 times better at a given duration of infertility. With respect to the age factor, the prognosis is lower by 9 per cent for each further year of the female partner's age. If a couple has primary infertility of four years' duration, and the female partner is 36 years of age, the likelihood of pregnancy is 25 per cent. If the female partner were 26 years of age, the prognosis would be 1.7 times, or 43 per cent, better.

Although this attempt to summarize the prognosis for unexplained infertility is based on data, it must be clear that such data cannot embrace the complexity of the clinical, personal, and social issues that may effect the various outcomes among such couples.

13 The emotional needs of the infertile couple

The earlier sections of this book have tried to arrive at a technical definition of unexplained infertility. It was proposed that the definition of infertility must be expanded from the simple time-linked 'inability to conceive' to encompass the deeply felt needs of the couple. Attention to these needs is no less the responsibility of the physician than attention to purely technical matters.

Aside from the obvious desire for a child, infertile couples will require support during the investigation and management. If a pregnancy cannot be achieved, a need which cannot be gratified may at least be resolved to a level where it is no longer all-consuming. Simply stated, the goals of the emotional management of the infertile couple will be to provide:

(1) support during the active phase of investigation and management; and

(2) assistance to face uncertainty or childlessness, if such are to be probable outcomes.

In order to achieve these goals, it is necessary to consider the emotional impact of infertility and to devise treatment strategies. This chapter will address:

(1) the research evidence;

(2) the emotional impact of infertility;

(3) support during investigation and management; and

(4) help in facing uncertainty or childlessness.

RESEARCH EVIDENCE

The relationship between psychosocial problems and infertility has been examined in various research protocols which have evaluated causation and interventions. Emotional and social problems may be linked with infertility, but whether causation exists in either direction has not been convincingly demonstrated (Wright *et al.* 1989). There are limitations both in experimental designs and in the precision of the definitions used for the purpose of discussing infertility. If there are emotional and behavioural influences that can cause infertility, it is reasonable to expect these influences to be measurably different among couples with unexplained infertility. While studies have long supported the conclusion that infertile couples are more psychosocially distressed that control groups (Mai *et al.* 1972), the distress may well be arising from the fact of the infertility, rather than causing the state of infertility (Lalos *et al.* 1985). Wright *et al.* (1989) conclude that the impact of infertility may be attenuated through psychosocial treatment; but the evidence is inconclusive and based mainly on poorly controlled outcome studies. No studies to date have addressed the question whether psychosocial interventions may help infertile couples through their psychosocial impact, or through the regaining of control that may follow from the acquisition of further knowledge about infertility.

EMOTIONAL IMPACT OF INFERTILITY

Infertility is frequently referred to as a 'crisis' (Menning 1982). Given the protracted nature of investigation and management, such a term can be misleading, suggesting as it does an immediate turning-point for better or for worse. Of the four definitions of crisis offered by Webster (1983), only one—'an unstable or crucial time or state of affairs in which a decisive change is impending; *esp.* one with the distinct possibility of a highly undesirable outcome' gives some sense of the prolonged nature of the stresses suffered by infertile couples. Even this definition implies that 'a decisive change is impending'. Such is rarely the situation of the infertile couple.

Their emotional life tends to be a prolonged roller-coaster, with periods of hope alternating with despair. Menning (1982) has characterized the stages through which most couples will progress. These include: surprise, denial, isolation, and guilt. For those who do not achieve pregnancy, resolution can only come after a period of grieving.

Individual men and women respond differently, both as members of a specific couple and as one individual person from another. A few seem to regard their infertility as simply another of life's vicissitudes, which can be dealt with and resolved rapidly. Such individuals are rare. At the other end of the spectrum, a small number of patients will exhibit frank symptoms of overtly psychiatric disorders, of which severe depression is the most prevalent (Seastrunk *et al.* 1984). It is probable that overt psychiatric illness is no more prevalent among infertile couples than among the general population; but such patients will require formal psychiatric help.

The great majority of patients do suffer from a greater or lesser degree of psychological distress, which will vary in intensity depending on their socio-economic background, the stage of investigation or treatment reached, the duration of their infertility, their age, their religious affiliations, and whether they are female or male (Daniluk 1988).

Once the period of surprise and denial have passed, the couple must deal with a plethora of conflicting feelings. The infertility represents a threat to attainment of one of life's goals, and may greatly tax their usual strategies for coping (Frank 1984; Seibel and Taymor 1982). Feelings of helplessness and desperation are common (Frank 1984). A sense of personal failure (Sawatzky 1981; Seibel and Taymor 1982) frequently commingles with feelings of guilt (Honea-Fleming and Honea 1984; Menning 1982). Such guilt may be related to previous events, including pre-marital sex, previous abortion or children surrendered for adoption, masturbation, and the derivation of pleasure from the sexual act (Griffin 1983; Menning 1982).

Self-esteem may suffer, with severe loss of self-image (Rosenfeld and Mitchell 1979). While the female partner often reveals her feelings, in Western society men are expected to be calm and unemotional. The potentially devastating effect upon the male psyche was demonstrated in one study where 63 per cent of men recently informed of their sterility became impotent for periods varying from one to three months (Berger 1980).

These emotional aspects can be manifested by symptoms of depression in over 80 per cent of both males and females (Seastrunk *et al*. 1984), hostility, and agitation (Seibel and Taymor 1982; Griffin 1983). Tension headaches, dyspepsia, sleep disorders, and exhaustion may all be experienced (Menning 1982).

Sexual function may be significantly affected, although a study of 500 couples (Menning 1982) failed to reveal any more sexual dysfunction among infertile couples than in fertile couples. The joy of sex can too readily become the job of sex, particularly when great emphasis is placed upon strict adherence to sexual scheduling. This may be self-inflicted, encouraged by well-meaning friends and self-help books, or, more frequently, may result from medical advice. The lack of value of timed mid-cycle coitus has been described. One particularly stressful procedure of strictly limited value is the post-coital test, the stressfulness of which has been described by Harrison (1981) and Drake and Grunert (1979). As many as 10 per cent of infertile couples describe some degree of mid-cycle sexual dysfunction (Drake and Grunert 1979).

Not surprisingly, great stress can be placed upon the relationship. Although the experience of infertility may actually strengthen interpersonal ties (Daniluk 1988), there may be specific difficulties related to communication, sexual activity, and the ability to plan together for the future (Mahlstedt 1985; Spencer 1987; Farrer-Meschan 1971). If a definite aetiology has been identified, the non-affected partner may question the attractiveness and value of the spouse (Menning 1977). Failure to communicate is frequent (Feuer 1983).

Clearly a great amount of distress is suffered. The feelings experienced will vary depending on where the couple is on the road of investigation, diagnosis, and management.

Daniluk (1988) sheds light on these issues from data based on a longitudinal study of 43 couples suffering from primary infertility. The couples were evaluated by questionnaire at the time of the initial visit, four weeks later during testing, within one week of diagnosis, and six weeks after the diagnosis had been made. Scores for psychological distress, relationship change, marital adjustment, and sexual satisfaction were derived from the questionnaires. This information, after submission to extensive univariate and multivariate analysis of dependence, was used to determine if changes occurred for both men and women, at which points during the investigation changes were most marked, and the nature of the changes. In addition, the impact of the diagnosis and the time spent in trying to conceive were studied.

The most important findings were that sexual satisfaction and marital adjustment did not seem to change significantly across the four testing sessions, and could not be related to the sex of the respondent, diagnostic information, identified aetiological source, or the time spent trying to conceive.

Psychological distress was greatest in both men and women at the time of the initial visit ($p \leqslant 0.05$). Higher levels of symptomatic psychological distress were observed in female participants than in male subjects at the time of diagnosis ($p \leqslant 0.07$). A diagnosis which explained the infertility was a cause of greater distress, particularly depression, than when the infertility was unexplained ($p \leqslant 0.05$).

Daniluk concluded: 'while the infertility investigation did not generally appear to result in extreme or incapacitating distress for the men and women in the study, the participants did appear to be experiencing a degree of symptomatic psychological distress as they proceeded through the various stages of the investigation'. Studies such as these serve to confirm an additional need for support during the time of investigation and treatment.

Two other phenomena are frequently described by infertile couples —feelings of isolation and helplessness (Daniluk 1988) and feelings of lack of any control (Lalos *et al.* 1985; Link and Darling 1986). This lack of control can be particularly frustrating, and may be the wellspring from which flows much of the psychological distress in infertile couples.

SUPPORT DURING THE ACTIVE PHASE OF INVESTIGATION AND MANAGEMENT

The principles of providing emotional support to the infertile couple during the active phase of investigation and management should include the recognition of:

(1) the times of greatest stress (the first visit, and the time of diagnosis);

(2) the inevitability of hostility and anger, often directed against the physician, and the need not to reply in kind;

(3) the fear of the unknown and the feelings of lack of control, which constitute perhaps the greatest stressors;

(4) the feelings of isolation; and

(5) the fact that a few patients will display symptoms of overt psychiatric disorders.

Few physicians will have formal training in counselling. This should inhibit no one from treating another human being with empathy, respect, and sensitivity to their needs.

As it is recognized that the first visit is one of the most stressful, an information package sent to the patients before this visit may help to allay some of the patients' fears. Both partners must be seen together. If necessary, individual appointments can be arranged later. Once the routine history and necessary physical examination have been performed, the needs of each individual couple should be established. The simple question 'What would you like us to do for you?' can elicit some surprising answers. To deal with the fear of the unknown, the specific investigative strategy must be discussed with the couple, and decisions whether or not to proceed with a given test or treatment option must be left to them. In this way, control is maintained by the couple. Whereas great comfort is derived by most people when a clear logical strategy has been decided upon, great distress can result from a disorganized approach. This process is described by Menning (1982) as 'planning together'.

As the investigation proceeds, ample time must be available to answer the inevitable questions which will arise, and simply to permit patients to express their hurt and confusion. In many clinics, these services are provided by the nursing staff.

A formal education programme, which describes the patho-physiology, causes and treatment of infertility, and allows sufficient time for discussion, may be beneficial. Subjects which might be discussed include the impact of infertility on life-style and the couple's relationship and coping mechanisms. Particular attention must be paid to the process of decision-making and mechanisms for maintaining control over the decision-making process. That people sometimes hear only what they want to hear was clearly demonstrated by a comparison of patient- versus-physician-rated prognosis (Taylor and McEwan 1986). Twenty-four per cent of women advised about the probability that tubal reparative surgery would succeed (in percentage terms) answered a questionnaire with responses suggesting that they simply had not processed the information. Their expectations were considerably greater than the objective facts expressed by the physician.

Support when a diagnosis of unexplained infertility has been made

Following the diagnosis of unexplained infertility the couple must face a considerable amount of uncertainty. Treatment-independent pregnancy may occur at any time. Many couples are driven by a need to 'do something' and, at this point, are very vulnerable to modern versions of the 'useless and injurious practice' referred to in 1883 by Matthews Duncan (quoted at the start of the Introduction to the present volume). At this time it is critical to work together towards a management strategy which, like the investigations, is clearly defined.

The therapeutic options, the risks, and the probable outcomes must be discussed. The couple must be actively involved with the decisions about when to start a particular regime and, more importantly, when to close the door on an unsuccessful option. This approach ensures that control remains with the couple, and permits many couples to satisfy their need to exert every reasonable effort on their own behalf. In order to facilitate this decision-making, the physician must clearly know the numerical probabilities that a given approach will or will not succeed. The physician must provide accurate data to help couples decide beforehand how long they will try a given treatment (Taylor 1990).

The role of other professionals

Many clinics provide the services of counsellors trained in the behavioural sciences. In some clinics, attendance for counselling is mandatory; in others, it is offered to patients in whom a need is perceived by the physician or the patients. Daniluk (1988) noted that 95 per cent of men and 90 per cent of women studied felt that the provision of such services would have helped to meet their needs. Nevertheless, among the same subjects, only 53 per cent of males and 72 per cent of females would personally have availed themselves of such services.

In one study, although 212 couples were offered counselling, only 62 attended (Bresnick and Taymor 1979). Of the attenders, only 50 per cent reported that the counselling had effected a positive change. Group therapy (Abarbanel and Bach 1959; Lukse 1985) is reported to be of value when the group is directed by a trained person. A behavioural approach to stress-reduction was also reported to reduce anxiety and improve fertility, but this study lacked a control group (Domar *et al.* 1990). In a small randomized study, fertility was improved in a group that received a psychological interview, but no cause-and-effect relationship was shown (Sarrel and DeCherney 1985). Many self-help support groups are available, which may help couples to deal with their feelings of isolation by allowing them to meet and converse with others in the same predicament.

No treatment, physical or psychological, is necessarily free of side-effects. The technical matters dealt with in this text have been submitted to intense scrutiny. Regrettably, the effects of counselling, individual, group, or self-help, have not. While it is not our intent to deny that infertile couples do have deeply felt needs, consistency demands that research should be urgently pursued to assess the efficacy of counselling.

Is it possible that the benefits perceived by some couples represent the healing effects of the passage of time rather than the effects of counselling? Is it possible that resolution of the conflict can be delayed by well-meaning advice from a member of a self-help group who has just heard about another miracle cure? We will continue to offer counselling services and suggest that patients attend self-help groups, and will await eagerly the publication of the results of such inquiries.

ASSISTANCE TO FACE UNCERTAINTY OR CHILDLESSNESS

Thus far, this chapter has addressed the first goal, that of support during active investigation and management. What of the second goal, that of assisting couples to face uncertainty and possible childlessness once all reasonable avenues have been exhausted? Attention to the principles described here—provision of accurate information, empathetic support, vesting control in the couple, and helping them to feel that they have indeed made their very best effort—may be the foundations of ultimate resolution. Such couples must be helped to feel not that they have 'given up' (a very negative statement in our society), but rather that they have done their very best and that they may now give themselves permission to let go.

Glazer and Cooper (1988) have suggested a practical list of questions that may help such couples define their feelings. These questions are:

1. How important is it to us to have a biological child versus no child or an adopted child?

2. How much longer can we tolerate the uncertainty of whether we will conceive a child?

3. How much more physical pain and risk can we take?

4. Are we willing to continue to have our daily routine interrupted by necessary medical tests and regimens?

5. To what extent has our relationship been negatively affected by infertility?

6. Can we afford (and do we choose) to spend more money on potentially expensive treatments?

CONCLUSIONS

The emotional needs of the infertile couple must be taken into consideration, no less than the purely technical. This chapter has discussed these needs and suggested some approaches by which, at least in part, they can be met.

14 Empirical treatments for unexplained infertility

INTRODUCTION

Once a diagnosis of unexplained infertility has been made, by definition no specific cause has been identified, and therefore no specific therapy to correct a causative defect is available. Even so, both couples and physicians find that they are under the greatest pressure to take some action. History abounds with examples of responses to this imperative, many of which fell under the heading of '. . . useless and injurious practice', to employ the language used by Matthews Duncan in 1883 (quoted at the start of the Introduction to this book). Few of these historical treatments had any basis in logic, and the same could be said for many of today's regimens. Nevertheless, a choice does exist between no active intervention and treatments which, although non-specific, do at least have a logical rationale, and may be associated with improved fertility. While the technical concerns are relatively straightforward, difficult decisions must be made. The first is to choose between treatment and no treatment. If the choice is made to treat, the timing of the treatment and the choice of individual treatment are also problematic, and will be dependent on decisions which should be made by the couple with the guidance of the physician. The next chapter will deal with the effectiveness of non-specific treatment; and the final chapter addresses the process of decision-making. This chapter will describe the rationale and technical aspects of such treatments.

The principle underlying all methods of treatment of unexplained infertility that are currently believed to be logical is to increase the mathematical chances of conception by increasing the number of oocytes that may be fertilized in a single cycle. By increasing the number of embryos, the chances of successful implantation appear to be improved. These ends may be achieved by ovarian stimulation and/or by bringing spermatozoa into closer proximity to mature oocytes. While the principle is relatively simple, a bewildering array of methods exists for its application. These include ovarian stimulation by an ever-expanding number of regimens, placing the spermatozoa within the uterus or fallopian tube, and the more technologically complex *in vitro* methods. The latter include *in vitro* fertilization and embryo transfer (IVF), gamete intrafallopian transfer (GIFT), zygote intrafallopian transfer (ZIFT), and pro-nuclear stage oocyte transfer (PROST). Each will be discussed in turn.

TECHNICAL ASPECTS

Ovarian stimulation

In any natural menstrual cycle, one or two mature oocytes will be released. For each oocyte, there is a probability that it will successfully enter the fallopian tube and be fertilized, and that the resultant embryo will survive and implant. It seems, at least at first sight, reasonable to postulate that if a larger number of oocytes is released the chances of one's being successfully fertilized should improve (Fisch *et al.* 1989). The hypothesis should hold true whether the spermatozoa are introduced into the female genital tract by natural or by artificial means. It is also postulated that if subtle defects of follicular or luteal development exist, use of exogenous agents might correct these defects (Daly 1989).

There are many protocols for ovarian stimulation. The agents most commonly used in these protocols are:

(1) clomiphene citrate;

(2) human menopausal gonadotrophins;

(3) gonadotrophin-releasing hormone agonists; and

(4) human chorionic gonadotrophin.

Clomiphene citrate

Clomiphene is a triphenyl chloroethylene derivative. Biologically, it is a non-steroidal oestrogen chemically similar to tamoxifen and chlorotrianisene (TACE). It is devoid of any significant oestrogenic, androgenic, or progestational effects in the human. Clomiphene is water-soluble, absorbed when given orally, and predominantly cleared by the liver and excreted in the faeces. About half the dose is cleared within five days, although residual traces may be found in the faeces several weeks later.

Clomiphene is active at the oestrogen receptors in the hypothalamus, pituitary, ovary, and uterus. Binding to these receptors effects competitive antagonism with oestrogen (Adashi 1984). The predominant effect is to produce a net increase in the secretion and release of follicle-stimulating hormone and luetinizing hormone, with resultant follicular recruitment. In the ovulatory patient (which would include those with unexplained infertility), subsequent events are driven by the developing follicles, leading to a mid-cycle luteinizing hormone surge and ovulation.

Patients with unexplained infertility are usually given doses of 50 to 100 mg per day (Fisch *et al*. 1989; Forsey and Hull 1989). Administration can begin anywhere from day two to day five of the cycle, and the usual course of treatment is five days. As the response to clomiphene is usually predictable, extensive monitoring of follicular development is not usually required. If more accurate timing of ovulation is desired, one or two ultrasonographic follicular scans may be performed, and ovulation may be triggered with a single injection of human chorionic gonadotrophin.

Clomiphene citrate is relatively free from side-effects. Of 8029 clomiphene cycles studied, ovarian enlargement was noted in 13.6 per cent, vasomotor flushes in 10.4 per cent, visual symptoms in 1.5 per cent, and acute abdominal symptoms in 0.2 per cent (Kistner 1975). The most frequent reasons for discontinuing the medication are the symptoms of diplopia and vasomotor flushes (Fisch *et al*. 1989; Hecht *et al*. 1989; Shalev *et al*. 1989). Detailed reviews of clomiphene citrate and its pharmacology and clinical application are provided by Corenblum and Taylor (1987) and Adashi (1984).

Human menopausal gonadotrophins

The urine of post-menopausal women contains high levels of the pituitary gonadotrophins luteinizing hormone (LH) and follicle-stimulating hormone (FSH). Kaolin extracts from pooled meno-pausal urine contain comparable amounts of LH and FSH (Borth *et al.* 1954). The gonadotrophins are glycoproteins with a molecular weight between 16 000 and 68 000 Daltons. Human menopausal gonadotrophins (HMG) are supplied in ampules containing 75 i.u. of FSH and 75 i.u. of LH activity.

The physiological actions whereby the gonadotrophins induce follicular recruitment and maturation have been described in detail in Chapter 3. In a natural cycle, one follicle will gain dominance while the others undergo atresia. The effect of the administration of exogenous gonadotrophins is to increase the number of follicles which continue to grow rather than undergo atresia. Numerous protocols of HMG administration are available and include those in which an initial dose of clomiphene is used to initiate follicular recruitment, those where HMG is used alone, and those where HMG and a gonadotrophin-releasing hormone agonist are used in combination (see later).

Until recently, the most commonly used approaches for women with unexplained infertility involved administration of HMG, 2 or 3 ampoules, by daily deep intramuscular injection, starting between day 2 and day 4 of the cycle (Daly 1989; Dodson *et al.* 1987; Serhal *et al.* 1988; Welner *et al.* 1988). Intensive monitoring of follicular development was performed using serial oestradiol and ultrasonic follicular measurements. Ovulation may occur following a spon-taneous LH surge, or may be induced by a single injection of human chorionic gonadotrophin.

The use of HMG is expensive, time-consuming, and not without risk. The major risks are ovarian hyperstimulation and multiple pregnancy. Mild ovarian hyperstimulation will occur in 31 to 60 per cent of cycles, and severe manifestations may be noted in 0.25 to 1.8 per cent of cycles (Lunenfeld and Lunenfeld 1990). The frequency of ovarian hyperstimulation, which fortunately is usually mild, is 7 per cent when HMG is used in the treatment of unexplained infertility (Dodson *et al.* 1987; Welner *et al.* 1988). Severe hyperstimulation results in massive ovarian enlargement and fluid shifts from the vascular compartment to the peritoneal and pleural cavities.

When HMG is used in anovulatory patients, the overall multiple pregnancy rate is 20 to 30 per cent (Gemzell 1977; Marshall 1970).

Of these, the majority are twins, but high-multiple pregnancies can occur despite intensive monitoring (Fedorkow *et al.* 1988).

Gonadotrophin-releasing hormone agonists

Gonadotrophin-releasing hormone (GnRH) is a decapeptide, the actions of which in the control of ovulatory function have been described in Chapter 5. Substitutions at positions six, nine, and ten produce powerful agonists whose initial action is similar to that of the natural GnRH, inducing a burst of LH release from the pituitary. Subsequently, the LH stored within the pituitary is depleted and, further, the receptors for GnRH on the pituitary gonadotrophs are down-regulated. Thus, subsequent release of LH is temporarily abolished (Clayton *et al.* 1982). Once the medication has been discontinued, normal LH secretion will resume within 7 to 14 days (Sandow *et al.* 1986).

While the agonists cannot by themselves induce ovulation, they do offer certain advantages. The initial release of LH can be used to recruit a cohort of follicles. These follicles can then be supported with HMG. As further endogenous release of LH has been abolished, ovulation will not occur spontaneously, but must be triggered by an injection of HCG. The loss of the spontaneous LH surge significantly reduces the amount of monitoring required.

The agonists are given by subcutaneous injection (Lewinthal *et al.* 1988) or intranasally (Sandow *et al.* 1986). A representative example of this class of compounds has a half life in serum of 80 minutes. Excretion is primarily in the form of inactive metabolites, 64 per cent of which appear in the urine and 12 per cent in the bile. A further 24 per cent is excreted intact in the urine (Sandow *et al.* 1986).

Three basic approaches to the use of GnRH agonists as adjuncts to induction of ovulation are in current clinical practice. Down-regulation with total abolition of LH activity may be started in the luteal phase (on day 23) of the preceding cycle, or on the second day of the follicular phase (Serafini *et al.* 1988). The third approach simply uses the known effect of the initial release of gonadotrophins after administration of the agonist to prompt follicular recruitment (Macnamee *et al.* 1989). The hold-over effect of down-regulation ensures that no spontaneous LH surge occurs, nor are there elevated tonic LH levels. The medication is given for three days, from the second to the fourth day of the cycle inclusive. Three ampoules of HMG are given from the third day of the menstrual cycle until the date of administration of human chorionic gonadotrophin.

There are essentially no side-effects attributable to the agonist using these protocols. The menopausal symptoms noted when these compounds are used in the long-term suppression of ovarian function for the treatment of endometriosis are attributable to oestrogen deficiency (Lemay *et al.* 1988). Such deficiency does not develop in patients undergoing induction of ovulation.

Human chorionic gonadotrophin

Human chorionic gonadotrophin is a glycoprotein which shares a common alpha subunit with FSH and LH, but differs in the beta subunit. Its major biological actions of interest when considering the induction of ovulation are its ability to mimic the mid-cycle LH surge, thus triggering ovulation, and its luteotrophic properties. To trigger ovulation, 5000 to 10 000 i.u. are administered intramuscularly when the follicle is judged to be mature (see later). Two thousand i.u. may be given at 3-day intervals post-ovulation to support the corpus luteum (Fisch *et al.* 1989).

Monitoring of induction or timing of ovulation

Rapid radio-immunoassay for oestradiol and ultrasound imaging of follicular development, particularly transvaginal ultrasonography, have greatly simplified the monitoring of the induction and timing of ovulation. Using any of the previously described agents (other than the simple administration of clomiphene citrate, where intensive monitoring is not required), the principles are identical. It is not the purpose of this chapter to describe in detail the plethora of available approaches, which seems to be as legion as the number of clinics providing such services. It would be impossible to do so. The principles only will be addressed.

Monitoring and timing hinge upon the recognition that an average mature follicle will produce approximately 500 pmol/l of oestradiol, and that follicles of diameters in excess of 15 mm will respond to exogenous HCG by release of a mature oocyte within 34 to 38 hours of the injection. The monitoring techniques in use should reduce cost and inconvenience to a minimum while still being accurate and safe. It is usual to administer the induction agent for a fixed number of days, at which time an oestradiol value will be measured. Based upon local laboratory values and programme experience, decisions will be made with respect to HMG dosage and when next to resort either to ultrasonographic or endocrine evaluation. Depending upon the indication for induction of ovulation, individual units will have established criteria whereby treatment may be cancelled, either because of a poor follicular response or because an exaggerated response carries too great a risk of hyperstimulation.

For those patients in whom follicular development is proceeding satisfactorily, ovulation will be induced with HCG when the dominant follicle is between 16 and 18 mm in diameter, and the total oestradiol is equal to or greater than 500 pmol/l times the number of follicles greater than 15 mm in diameter. Couples attempting to achieve pregnancy using spontaneous intercourse are instructed to do so 12 to 48 hours after HCG administration (Serhal *et al*. 1988; Welner *et al*. 1988).

The principles of induction of ovulation described in this section, which can be used in association with natural intercourse for couples with unexplained infertility, are also those used in conjunction with intrauterine or intratubal insemination of prepared spermatozoa or with one of the IVF variants. These treatments will now be addressed.

Intrauterine and intratubal insemination

The rationale for the use of intrauterine insemination for unexplained infertility is to place spermatozoa in closer juxtaposition with the oocyte, in the hope that some unidentified defect in sperm transport will be overcome.

Jansen *et al*. (1988) and Brooks *et al*. (1988) have placed the spermatozoa directly within the fallopian tubes using either ultrasonically-guided catheters or hysteroscopically-placed catheters. Attempts to achieve successful pregnancy have been made both in natural ovulatory cycles and in conjunction with programmes of controlled ovarian hyperstimulation. It is apparent that simple intrauterine placement of spermatozoa in natural cycles does not produce any therapeutic benefit (Glass and Ericsson 1978; Nachtigall *et al*. 1979). There is increasing interest in the combination of controlled ovarian hyperstimulation combined with supracervical placement of spermatozoa. In such cycles of treatment, a stimulation of ovulation protocol using human menopausal gonadotrophins is instituted and ovulation is accurately timed. Insemination is performed with prepared spermatozoa using a fine transfer catheter, which is passed through the external cervical os to the interior of the uterine cavity. Whether single or multiple insemination should be carried out is as yet unknown. Programmes performing one insemination usually do so about 38 hours after the ovulation-triggering injection of HCG (Dodson and Haney 1991; teVelde *et al*. 1989).

Raw semen cannot be placed directly within the uterine cavity, as the seminal prostaglandins may cause violent intrauterine contraction, leading to vasovagal collapse. If intrauterine insemination is to be performed, spermatozoa must first be prepared by removing the spermatozoa from the seminal plasma. It is the aim of the sperm-penetration techniques to isolate the most fertile fraction of the ejaculate. Approaches currently in use include:

(a) simple sperm-wash methods;

(b) migration or swim-up methods;

(c) washing, centrifugation, and swim-up; and

(d) the use of discontinuous gradient separation techniques.

Simple sperm-washing

Simple sperm-washing involves dilution of the liquefied semen with medium, centrifugation at low speed, and resuspension of the sperm pellet in the medium. While this method eliminates the deleterious effects of the seminal plasma, all the sperm, including those which are immotile and any particulate or bacteriological matter, will be included in the material to be inseminated. It is also possible that poor-quality spermatozoa, by generating free oxygen radicals, may be harmful to other spermatozoa in the preparation.

Migration swim-up methods

This modification of the original approach to sperm preparation for IVF involves layering media over the spermatozoa and waiting 30 to 60 minutes. The upper, or 'buffy', coat is removed. This approach will yield a higher percentage of motile sperm (Wiltbank *et al*. 1985).

Washing, centrifugation, and swim-up

The simple swim-up technique has been refined by the use of a one- or two-step wash and centrifugation with swim-up recovery, and is associated with the successful recovery of relatively high numbers of motile sperm and little debris.

The use of discontinuous gradient separation techniques

A discontinuous gradient of Percoll can be used to enhance recovery of motile sperm. Nycodenz is an iodinated organic molecule dissolved in a tris buffer, which is biologically inert and non-toxic. A recent comparative study of Nycodenz with Percoll has shown Nycodenz gradients to be superior in separating a highly motile fraction of sperm (Gellert-Mortimer *et al*. 1988).

Given the rapid growth of techniques of sperm preparation, it is difficult to define the best. On the basis of current data, the use of Percoll and Nycodenz will probably result in harvesting the highest concentration of motile spermatozoa.

Once insemination has been performed, it is customary to support the luteal phase with either human chorionic gonadotrophin injections or pure progesterone if the stimulation protocol has involved the use of a GnRH agonist (Herman *et al*. 1990; Buvat *et al*. 1988). The efficacy of these agents, if the controlled ovarian stimulation has not used an agonist, is questionable (Crosignani *et al*. 1988; Hutchinson-Williams *et al*. 1990).

In vitro fertilization (IVF) and its variants

Since the birth of Louise Brown in 1978 (Steptoe and Edwards 1978), there has been an explosion in the application of *in vitro* fertilization techniques. While initially used for the treatment of tubal infertility, *in vitro* fertilization was rapidly applied to cases of unexplained infertility. An extensive review of these advanced reproductive technologies is beyond the scope of this chapter. Their principles will be described.

The most common approach is in its first part similar to the controlled ovarian hyperstimulation regimen described earlier in this chapter. Most clinical services now use a combination of GnRH agonists and human menopausal gonadotrophins. Monitoring and timing of impending ovulation are carried out in the same fashion. Historically, the mature oocytes were aspirated from the follicles by laparoscopically directed puncture. This method of oocyte pick-up was soon replaced by transabdominal and, more recently, transvaginal ultrasound-guided follicular aspiration. Once the oocytes have been identified, they are incubated with previously prepared spermatozoa. The methods of sperm preparation, once again, are variable, and are essentially similar to those described for intrauterine insemination.

The embryos which develop are cultured for about 36 to 48 hours and then replaced within the uterine cavity through a transcervical transfer catheter. This, then, in principle, is *in vitro* fertilization and embryo transfer (IVF). In order to improve the chances of successful conception, excess embryos may be cryopreserved and stored for replacement in a subsequent natural cycle.

Dissatisfied with the relatively poor success rate of IVF, Asch *et al.* (1986) introduced gamete intrafallopian transfer (GIFT). In contradistinction to IVF, the oocytes and sperm are returned to the fallopian tube, so that fertilization and early embryonic development will occur in the natural environment. Until recently, access to the tube required that laparoscopy should be performed—a much more invasive procedure than transvaginal oocyte recovery. Reports are now appearing of the successful placement of oocytes that were recovered transvaginally and prepared spermatozoa in the ampulla of the tube by ultrasonographically-guided transcervical catheterization. GIFT has the advantage of being ethically acceptable to some religious groups, in as much as fertilization does not occur outside the body. This is also its drawback. If a successful pregnancy does not occur, no insight has been gained into the process of fertilization.

To observe early embryonic development, and in attempts further to improve the success rate, intrauterine transfers of pre-embryos at both the pro-nuclear stage (PROST) and zygotic stage (ZIFT) have been undertaken. At present, it is not possible to state whether these variations are more successful and will replace GIFT, or will simply become interesting footnotes in the history of the assisted reproductive technologies.

Although all the empirical methods—controlled ovarian hyperstimulation, controlled ovarian hyperstimulation plus supracervical placement of spermatozoa, and IVF and its variants—have been used to treat couples with unexplained infertility, their true place in the therapeutic armamentarium has not been fully established. The place of any therapy depends on the ratio of its effectiveness to its known drawbacks, including costs, side-effects, and risks. The next chapter will deal with the effectiveness of treatment for unexplained infertility; and, in a final chapter, the process of decision-making with respect to the individual couple will be discussed.

15 An evaluation of empirical treatment of unexplained infertility

INTRODUCTION

Medical practice is more successful and more satisfying when rational, effective therapy to correct specific defects is available, particularly if such therapy leads to a desirable outcome. As, by definition, no specific defect can be identified in patients with unexplained infertility, there can be no rationale for therapy. We can only guess as to which of the many underlying reproductive mechanisms might be defective.

Well-designed clinical studies have the potential to exert the most powerful influence on effective clinical practice. The recent astounding growth in the use of electronic literature-searching indicates that patients' problems are increasingly likely to be resolved with the aid of published evidence. Decisions based on sound evidence are likely to lead to more effective treatment, or treatment which offers better efficiency or fewer side-effects. Where there is a choice, clinical protocols should be based upon the best available evidence. A key factor in the interpretation of clinical studies is the quality of the study design. It is the purpose of this chapter to discuss the design of studies for the evaluation of treatment, and to review and evaluate critically those studies which have been published about various empirical treatments of unexplained fertility.

STUDY DESIGN FOR THE EVALUATION OF TREATMENT

In any condition, such as infertility, where spontaneous cure is possible, the effect of treatment can only be judged by comparison

Table 15.1 *A comparison of steps in the design of trials for the evaluation of therapeutic efficacy*

Methodological considerations	Cohort studies	Randomized clinical trials
Eligibility criteria	Detailed specification	Detailed specification
Allocation method	Choice	Random
Manœuvre	Document treatment exposures	Document treatment exposures
Outcome definition	Specified in advance	Specified in advance

with the effect of no treatment. When the value of a treatment has been proved in this way, then later studies may compare new treatments with the now-standard treatment, rather than with a placebo treatment. Among such comparative studies, the randomized clinical trial is the most powerful design, because it minimizes bias. Statistical theory is based on the fundamental importance of chance in the allocation of the groups, and allocation by chance can exist only after randomization. Cohort studies are in a second class of quality, because treatment is chosen rather than allocated by chance; but even within this class of studies, better designs should reduce bias to a minimum. Table 15.1 shows an elementary comparison of these two study designs. Thus designing a cohort study can be as demanding as designing a randomized clinical trial. All clinical research will be more effective if the sample size is sufficiently large (the study has the power) to detect a difference, if one exists.

Cohort studies and randomized clinical trials will be discussed in detail in this chapter. An ineffective study design with respect to treatment efficacy is the uncontrolled case series. As uncontrolled reports dominate the literature on the treatment of unexplained infertility, some comment on these studies is necessary.

Uncontrolled studies

Because pregnancy occurs commonly among untreated infertile couples, comparison studies are needed to infer that the observed pregnancy rate is related to treatment. Nevertheless, many studies are simple case series, in which the earlier infertility is considered to serve as a control for treatment. Such case series may be useful in defining the proportion of side-effects and other events that may occur among individuals receiving treatment—although such events may have occurred by chance; but they cannot help us to understand the effect of treatment on fertility. In any group of subjects receiving treatment, the observed pregnancies can be attributed to the treatment only if a suitable untreated control group is available for comparison.

Because few comparative studies have been published, there is an unavoidable tendency to compare treated subjects reported in one study and untreated subjects reported elsewhere. Not surprisingly, pregnancy rates per cycle with treatment are generally superior to the observations among untreated groups. There are many reasons to reject the idea of comparing data derived from different sources. There may have been many months of observation in the untreated groups, compared with a few cycles of observation during treatment. Differences in the duration of infertility and other baseline prognostic factors affect the pregnancy rate, and these are often not defined. If a group of couples with infertility of short duration is treated, the pregnancy rate will inevitably be higher than that observed in a group with infertility of longer duration. The erroneous conclusion may then be drawn that the treatment has been effective.

An unexpected bias can arise from the seemingly innocent selection of patients according to some factor, such as treatment, that may affect the average length of follow-up. For example, the average duration of intensive treatment such as superovulation and intrauterine insemination is two to three months (Dodson and Haney 1991). Selecting couples according to their length of follow-up can affect the observed fecundity in unexpected ways, which are only explained after careful examination of the life-table observations for larger groups.

To illustrate this point, observations among 381 untreated couples with unexplained infertility, some of whom were followed for 48 months, were used to calculate the average monthly fecundability during months 1 to 6, and 7 to 12. The fecundability was approximately 4 per cent per month during the first six months, and 2 per cent per month during the second six months (Table 15.2). What is happening here is that when any group of infertile couples

Table 15.2 *Effect of selection according to the length of follow-up on fecundability among 381 untreated couples with unexplained infertility*

Selection criterion	Number of couples	Approximate fecundability (per cent per month)	
		1 to 6 months	7 to 12 months
All subjects	381	4.2	2.2
Followed up to 12 m only	202	11.4	11.1
Followed up to 6 m only	140	22.1	—

Data from the Canadian Infertility Therapy Evaluation Study (Vutyavanich and Collins 1991)

is assembled and observed, those who are more likely to get pregnant will conceive early in the observation period, and the proportion of pregnancies is much smaller in the remaining couples during later periods of observation.

This effect can be magnified enormously. When 202 of the original 381 patients were selected on the basis that they had been followed for no more than twelve months, the fecundability was 11 per cent. When the selection was made on the basis of an even shorter length of follow-up (6 months), the fecundability in this group of 140 couples was an astounding 22 per cent.

The single feature that emerges most clearly from an assessment of the uncontrolled studies on the treatment of unexplained infertility is the compelling need for comparative studies.

Cohort studies

Many comparative studies are not the product of random allocation. A group or 'cohort' of treated couples is compared with a group of untreated couples. Because the treated group have elected to have treatment or have been selected for treatment by their physicians, there will often be baseline differences between the groups which could bias the comparison of their pregnancy rates. Such cohort studies may be prospective studies, when the investigators set out the study methodology in advance and begin to recruit patients according to an explicit protocol. Retrospective cohort studies are also reported, when investigators similarly specify study methodology in advance, but go back in time to examine two separate groups of patient records which fulfil the eligibility criteria.

Sample specification

For a cohort study, a detailed definition of eligibility is required, with specific inclusion and exclusion criteria. The consecutive assembly of eligible subjects is more than usually important, in order to avoid the bias that arises from the informal exclusion of certain patients. A complete clinical description of the subjects is also essential, because it is very likely that the treatment groups will differ in fundamental ways, and these differences must be recorded. An estimate of the required sample size should be calculated, based on reasonable predictions of the expected differences between the groups, to be evaluated by conventional significance and power considerations. These sample-size considerations will be discussed here, although they apply equally to the design of randomized clinical trials.

Sample-size considerations

The required sample size is dependent upon both clinical and statistical considerations. The clinical considerations take into account the success associated with standard therapy, and require that the improvement with the new therapy is important enough to make a difference in clinical management. That difference is usually referred to as δ.

The first statistical consideration is the assumption about type I error (α), which allows for the possibility that the results with the new therapy might be better than the standard therapy purely by chance. This possibility is generally accepted in one of twenty trials ($\alpha = 0.05$).

Type II error (β), which is the error of not discovering a true difference when it exists, must also be considered. Conventional levels of β are usually set in the range of 0.1 to 0.2, so that the trial would have 90 per cent or 80 per cent power, respectively, to detect a true difference. In general, the sample-size requirement is increased by reductions in α, β, or δ, the clinical difference.

Manœuvre

As cohort studies take place in clinical practice settings, therapy decisions may be based on practice algorithms and upon patient needs and wishes. In order to document the exposure thoroughly, details of dosage, start and finish dates, compliance, and current medications are an essential part of the record, and should be available in reported studies.

Outcome

The results of cohort-analytic comparative studies are more convincing when the outcome is clear-cut and well defined. Nevertheless, even such an apparently clear event as pregnancy requires further definition. The choices include any clinical pregnancy (defined by tissue report, ultrasound, or delivery) and the alternative outcome, live birth.

Methods of analysis

Where the follow-up period is brief, and losses to follow-up are negligible, the comparison of simple pregnancy rates can serve as a satisfactory method of analysis. The comparison should be adjusted for the presence of baseline differences between the two groups in important prognostic variables such as the duration of infertility. In the case of simple pregnancy rates, the results may be expressed in the form of a two-by-two table, from which can be calculated the relative risk and the odds ratio (Table 15.3).

The relative risk is the most accurate estimate of the treatment effect; but many studies make use of the equally acceptable odds ratio. In either case, the result of the calculation is a single-point estimate of the true effect. The relative accuracy of the point-estimate is expressed by means of a 95 per cent confidence interval, and the confidence interval can be used to evaluate significance. Fig. 15.1 illustrates how the treatment effect can be expressed by means of the odds ratio with its confidence limits, expressing the odds of pregnancy with treatment compared with the odds of pregnancy without treatment. In study number one in this figure, there is no

Table 15.3 *Evaluation of studies on the efficacy of infertility treatment*

	Outcome Pregnant	Not pregnant
Group		
Treated	a	b
Untreated	c	d

$$\text{relative risk} = \frac{a}{a + b} \div \frac{c}{c + d}$$

$$\text{odds ratio} = ad \div bc.$$

apparent treatment effect. In study number two, there is a possible treatment effect, but the lower end of the confidence interval crosses the line representing unity, or no effect; thus the treatment may be promising, but the effect has not been proved with conventional statistical significance. In study number three, a treatment effect is observed and, in this case, the treatment effect has been proved.

Although simple pregnancy rates are useful to describe the clinical outcome in studies with relatively short periods of follow-up, with longer periods of follow-up couples may withdraw from observation or may become lost to follow-up. In order to allow for these events, and for the elapsed time prior to pregnancy occurring, survival analysis is usually required. These procedures were described in Chapter 12, and in general they evaluate the occurrence of an event such as pregnancy over a period of time, while adjusting for the effect of prognostic factors such as age, duration of infertility, and pregnancy history. The analysis also allows for events such as treatment that may arise in the course of follow-up. A multivariate approach is generally required for cohort studies, because it can adjust for the baseline differences that may be expected in the treated and untreated groups.

The strengths and weaknesses of cohort studies are summarized in

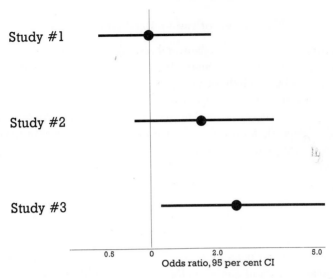

Fig. 15.1 *Graphic representation of treatment effects expressed by means of odds ratios with confidence limits.*

Table 15.4. Despite their strengths, the biases that arise from baseline differences and other sources create serious difficulties in the interpretation of the results of cohort studies. These difficulties can only be overcome by making use of designs which feature randomized allocation.

Table 15.4 *The strengths and weaknesses of cohort studies in the evaluation of therapeutic efficacy*

Strengths

10	The subjects are representative of clinical practice.
20	The selection is unbiased by trial protocols.
30	More than one treatment can be simultaneously evaluated.
40	All reasonable outcomes can be assessed.

Weaknesses

10	Crucial baseline differences are common.
20	Doctor and patient biases determine treatment.
30	There may be competing interventions in a single subject.
40	The treatment times and observation times are different.

The design of randomized clinical trials

The role of chance is a fundamental assumption in the application of statistical theory, and random allocation to treatment groups is the only means by which the play of chance can be ensured. Randomization is the key element of comparative study design, and the absence of randomization detracts from the credibility of any study. High-quality studies depend, however, on much more than just randomization. Careful attention must be paid to the assembly of groups, to the manœuvre itself, and to the definition of the outcome and its analysis.

Sample specification

Having defined the target population in a clear and specific way, the investigator should establish eligibility rules, with specific inclusion and exclusion criteria. These should be carefully developed in the light of the purpose of the trial. In explanatory trials which are designed to evaluate the efficacy of a single treatment in isolation from other influences, a group of similar subjects who are highly selected after careful screening would be desirable. Management trials should include more heterogeneous subjects who will be typical of infertile couples in general, in order to evaluate how effective the treatment would be in the average health-care setting.

The manœuvre

The process of randomization should be as free of bias as is practically possible. A random-number generator should be used, and ideally the allocation should be determined by telephone, or in some other way removed from the clinical-care setting. All other attempts to allow chance to determine allocation are open to systematic bias, and therefore the use of 'even versus odd' hospital numbers, alternate subjects, alternate days, and so on are not acceptable methods of randomization. The treatment itself should be exactly specified, and where possible placebo treatment should be used to avoid patient and observer bias. Double-binding is always preferable.

Outcome

At the beginning of the design process, the investigator must determine which specific outcome among the range of choices that usually exist will be defined as the primary outcome. Among infertility trials, pregnancy is the usual primary outcome, although live birth is sometimes a preferable alternative. In IVF protocols, the number of oocytes retrieved, the number of embryos transferred, or some other substitute outcome might be considered. Making such a choice accepts that there will be a reduction in the practical or clinical importance of the study. Such surrogate outcomes are important, and may contribute to our understanding of treatment and disease processes; but, for the purposes of clinical protocols, the outcome ideally should be that which is of primary interest to the clinical subject.

Methods of analysis

In the analysis, the question is put to the test. If the outcome is different in groups exposed to the alternative interventions, did this difference arise by chance, was it due to unintended maldistributions of prognostic factors in the groups, or is it possible to infer that there was a true difference between the two interventions (treatment and placebo)? Here again simple pregnancy rates or survival techniques with cumulative pregnancy rates can be used. The analysis may be univariate or, if baseline differences between the groups exist, multivariate.

Cross-over studies

The phrase 'randomized, cohort, double-blinded, cross-over trial' has come to be recognized as the gold standard of therapy trials. Cross-over designs were developed so that each patient receives both treatment and control, and they are most applicable where there is a considerable variability between patients, and less variability over time in the same patient. Thus cross-over designs reduce the effect of intrasubject variability, because the subjects serve as their own controls during each phase of the trial. They are most appropriate where there are short-term changes due to therapy, and when these changes are rapidly reversed (Petrie 1982). In studying an event such as pregnancy, however, any meaningful response withdraws the individual from the study, so that no intrasubject comparison is possible. Moreover, the withdrawal contributes to potentially serious imbalance between the groups under study. Table 15.5 illustrates how the effects of chance can be magnified in such cross-over designs.

In this example, two hypothetical groups of women with equal

Table 15.5 *The effect of a cross-over design on the occurrence of pregnancy during two exactly equal treatments*

Assumptions
1. Treatment a and treatment b are exactly equal with respect to pregnancy.
2. Group m (100 women) and group n (100 women) have equal fecundability.
3. The expected number of pregnancies during six months is 20 in each group.

Observations
1. During the first three months, there are 13 pregnancies in group m and seven in group n rather than the expected 20. This imbalance will occur by chance in approximately one in six trials.

2. After the cross-over, the imbalance within groups is corrected, and at the end of six months there are 20 pregnancies in both group m and group n, as expected.

3. There are $(13 + 13) = 26$ pregnancies with treatment a and $(7 + 7) = 14$ pregnancies with treatment b.

The analysis by treatment would be:

Treatment	Outcome Pregnant	Not pregnant	Total
a	26	74	100
b	14	86	100
Total	40	160	200

Statistic	Value	DF	Prob.
Pearson Chi Square	4.50	1	0.0339
Yates Corrected Chi Square	3.78	1	0.0518

fecundability are exposed to exactly equal treatments. By chance, a few more pregnancies occur in one group than in the other during the first period of observation. After the treatment cross-over, this chance imbalance is corrected, with the result that one treatment appears to be more effective than the other. Although the final result is due only to a chance occurrence, the chi square for the ensuing comparison of treatments is associated with a p value equal to 0.0518. It would take a very strong will indeed to resist calling treatment 'A' superior to treatment 'B' after such a trial; but in fact the treatments are, as they were before the trial, exactly equivalent.

In a less dramatic way, a similar bias arises from designs in which treatments are allocated by cycle, because subjects who conceive will not be exposed equally to each treatment. Given the degree of bias that can be created by the cross-over design in a randomized study, it can be seen how this error may be magnified in non-randomized studies, especially those where individuals who fail to conceive with one treatment are then given a second treatment, and the results with treatments one and two are subsequently compared. If there is an equivalent natural force of pregnancy in such patients, the last treatment given will usually seem better after the analysis of such studies.

Randomized clinical trials with cross-over designs may be inappropriate for the study of dichotomous and final end-points such as pregnancy; but it would be equally inappropriate to ignore the information in these otherwise well-designed studies. One approach is to evaluate the information derived from the pre-cross-over portion of the trial, when and if that information is reported. Where randomization is by cycle, however, the information for the first cycle is rarely reported as a separate experience. The information from retrospective studies with cross-over to a new treatment after failure of the 'control treatment' is virtually useless for comparative purposes.

By comparison with cohort studies, randomized clinical trials represent an elaborate and expensive method of evaluating therapy. Nevertheless, because randomization reduces bias, justifies the use of statistical methodology, and allows for concealment or blinding, the clinical audience in the 1990s will be more likely to base judgements about therapy on studies which are based on meticulously worked-out randomized designs.

Relevance and clinical significance

To be applicable in a clinical practice, published material should be relevant to the problems that are generally seen in such a practice, and it goes without saying that the reported treatment should be available for use. It is also important that the report should encompass subjects who are typical, and therefore will be similar to the average patient. Often subjects reported in studies from tertiary treatment centres have a much more severe form of any given disorder than those seen in everyday practice, and their outcomes after treatment may be quite different from those of other patients. Study results should arise from a persuasive study design, as has just been argued, and the results should have not only clinical but statistical significance. The concept of statistical significance is in common usage, and requires little explanation. It has come to be accepted that a probability of a chance result of less than 0.05 represents a result which is considered statistically significant, regardless of the test statistic on which the result is based. Conventionally, when the probability is less than 1 in 20 that the observed result much have arisen by chance, we are prepared to accept that an effect exists.

Clinical significance is also important. If, for example, a study of two *in vitro* fertilization protocols found that in one 4.6 oocytes were retrieved on average, while in the other a mean of 4.9 oocytes were retrieved, the difference might be highly significant. In practical terms, however, the observed difference would be of no importance to the individual patient, and only of marginal importance to protocol designers. Thus, in the interpretation of clinical results, both statistical and clinical significance should be taken into account.

These concepts of significance, together with an awareness of the quality of a given study design, and the clinician's intrinsic knowledge of the practicability of treatments, all combine to aid in applying published evidence in day-to-day clinical concerns.

EFFICACY OF REPORTED TREATMENT

In this section comparative studies of treatment for unexplained infertility are summarized. The treatments evaluated in such studies include bromocriptine, danazol, intrauterine insemination, clomiphene, menopausal gonadotrophins used alone or in conjunction with intrauterine insemination, and various *in vitro* techniques.

Bromocriptine

Three randomized trials of bromocriptine compared with placebo have revealed no measurable difference in observed pregnancy rates (Harrison *et al.* 1979; McBain and Pepperell 1982; Wright *et al.* 1979). These studies had relatively small sample sizes and limited power, and one of them was based on a cross-over design (McBain and Pepperell 1982). There have been no subsequent studies, and bromocriptine is for practical purposes no longer in favour as a non-specific therapy for unexplained infertility.

Bromocriptine treatment was further evaluated in patients with unexplained infertility and expressible galactorrhoea in a cohort study. The pregnancy rate was higher with bromocriptine therapy than with pyridoxine therapy (DeVane and Guzick 1986). In this study the controls were older, they had a longer duration of infertility, and their pre-treatment prolactin levels were lower than the pre-treatment concentrations in the bromocriptine-treated group. Thus, even in the presence of expressible galactorrhoea, the value of bromocriptine therapy as a treatment for unexplained infertility has not been satisfactorily proved because of the baseline differences in the groups.

Danazol

Two studies have evaluated danazol for the treatment of unexplained infertility (Iffland *et al.* 1989; Van Dijk *et al.* 1979). In the first of these, 5 of 21 danazol-treated patients conceived, compared with 1 of 19 placebo-treated controls, but 1 other control subject was excluded because of a conception that occurred within the six-month placebo-treated period. In the second study, there were no pregnancies among the 14 danazol-treated patients, and 1 in the control group. The expense of danazol, its prolonged contraceptive effect, and its lack of efficacy with respect to fertility, even in the treatment of endometriosis, all suggest that this drug is a poor choice.

Intrauterine insemination (IUI)

Intrauterine insemination with washed sperm has been advocated as a treatment for couples with unexplained infertility. Although promising, the treatment appears to have been accepted as therapeutically beneficial before evidence from adequately controlled studies was available to demonstrate its efficacy. Intrauterine insemination was first used for the treatment of male infertility, and the results of three comparative studies do not support its efficacy in the presence of oligoasthenozoospermia (Ho *et al*. 1989; Hughes *et al*. 1987; teVelde *et al*. 1989). An earlier study presented a different view (Kerin *et al*. 1984).

Two studies have evaluated intrauterine insemination as a treatment for unexplained infertility by means of a comparison with an untreated control group. Martinez *et al*. (1991) randomly allocated patients stratified by diagnosis to a balanced set of treatments arranged by cycle. In this study, among those with unexplained infertility, 3 pregnancies occurred in 33 intrauterine insemination cycles, and 1 occurred in 35 timed-intercourse cycles. Half of each group of cycles was stimulated with clomiphene, and the pregnancy rate with intrauterine insemination was not significantly superior.

Kirby *et al*. (1991) randomly allocated patients to a first cycle of intrauterine insemination or timed intercourse, and in subsequent cycles the treatments were alternated. Among 73 couples with unexplained infertility there were 6 pregnancies in 145 intrauterine insemination cycles, and 3 pregnancies in 123 cycles of timed intercourse, a difference which was not significant.

The results of these two studies individually and combined do not support the efficacy of intrauterine insemination for the treatment of unexplained infertility. The treatment does appear, however, to be reasonably safe. IUI treatment seems to be reasonably free of hazards, one of which could be an increase in the prevalence of anti-sperm antibodies. Recent evidence indicates that the intrauterine placement of prepared spermatozoa does not alter the frequency of anti-sperm antibody detected by immunobead assays (Goldberg *et al*. 1990; Horvath *et al*. 1989). Although the evidence is not conclusive, intrauterine insemination alone seems to have no proven benefit among couples with unexplained infertility. Better evidence on this point would be important, because intrauterine insemination is frequently used as the control treatment in studies evaluating superovulation protocols, some of which also include intrauterine insemination. Given the evidence to date, intrauterine insemination in such studies may serve, whether so intended or not, as a placebo treatment.

Clomiphene treatment

Clomiphene citrate is associated with a dose-dependent rise in the number of ovarian follicles, suggesting that the mechanism of clomiphene action in the treatment of unexplained infertility could be through a process of superovulation. There are now two trials of clomiphene therapy compared with placebo therapy for unexplained infertility, and a further trial in which clomiphene therapy combined with intrauterine insemination was compared with natural cycles and timed intercourse (Table 15.6) (Deaton *et al.* 1990; Fisch *et al.* 1989; Glazener *et al.* 1990).

In the first of these studies, women were randomly allocated to receive clomiphene or placebo tablets and luteal phase HCG or placebo injections for four months (Fisch *et al.* 1989). The study design evaluated four treatment groups (placebo/placebo, HCG/placebo, clomiphene/placebo, and HCG/clomiphene). As originally reported, the treated groups had a superior pregnancy rate, no pregnancies having been observed among 36 placebo-treated women during 4 cycles. In a re-analysis using a logistic regression method reported elsewhere, the HCG made no contribution to fertility

Table 15.6 *Randomized clinical trials evaluating clomiphene in the treatment of unexplained infertility*

Authors	Patients	Pregnancy per cycle (per cent) Treated	Control	Duration (months) of infertility
Deaton *et al.* 1990	51	8/73 (11.0)	4/103 (3.9)	42
Fisch *et al.* 1989	148	10/290 (3.5)	4/274 (1.5)	51
Glazener *et al.* 1990	118	24/108 (2.2)	15/105 (1.4)	28

(Collins 1990*b*). Thus the data summarized here comprise the experience among 76 clomiphene-treated women during 290 cycles (10 pregnancies) compared with 72 women who received the oral placebo during 274 cycles (four pregnancies).

In the second of these studies, 118 women with unexplained infertility were treated with clomiphene in a randomized placebo-controlled cross-over study in which women were assigned to 3 months with each preparation (Glazener *et al.* 1990). There were 24 clomiphene-associated pregnancies during 294 cycles, compared with 15 placebo-associated pregnancies during 295 cycles among women with 28 months duration of infertility whose average age was 28 years (Glazener *et al.* 1990). The experience of the subjects during the pre-cross-over period was not reported. In each of these two studies the dosage of clomiphene was 100 mg daily for five days.

In the third study, 51 couples entered a cross-over trial evaluating clomiphene citrate (50 mg) combined with intrauterine insemination in the treatment of 24 women with unexplained infertility and 27 with previously treated endometriosis (Deaton *et al.* 1990). The authors reported a statistically significant difference in fertility, as there were 14 pregnancies in 148 treated cycles, compared with 5 pregnancies in 150 untreated cycles. The experience prior to cross-over, however, included 8 pregnancies during 73 treatment cycles and four pregnancies during 103 control cycles, and this difference is not significant at the 5 per cent level. The data after cross-over may represent the bias demonstrated in Table 15.5.

The relative likelihood of pregnancy based on the results in the three studies is illustrated graphically in Fig. 15.2. Individually, each of the studies suggests that clomiphene increases the relative likelihood of pregnancy, although each confidence interval overlaps unity, so that the effect is not proven. The combined odds ratio shows the effect of clomiphene to be approximately twice that of a placebo.

When the results of different studies are combined in this way some measure is needed of the variability from study to study. If the individual study results are homogeneous or similar, the combined results would be more convincing than in the case where one study shows a positive effect and others are negative. In the latter case the results of the studies are heterogeneous. In testing for such variability

Authors

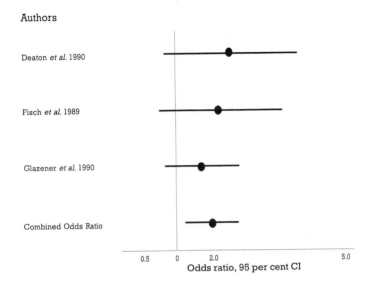

Fig. 15.2 *Relative likelihood of pregnancy with clomiphene treatment in unexplained infertility.*

it is preferable not to find a significant (*p* value less than 0.05) degree of heterogeneity.

The Breslow and Day (1980) statistical test in the clomiphene trials was associated with a *p* value of 0.94, indicating that the intra-study comparisons are far from being significantly heterogeneous. This statistical evidence of homogeneity is reassuring, in view of the different inclusion criteria (including patients with treated endometriosis in the case of Deaton *et al.* (1990)).

Selection of patients

The better fecundity with clomiphene does not appear to be related to the size of the lead follicle or the number of dominant follicles detected by ultrasound. The best dosage has yet to be established. In the three cited studies, two used 100 mg for 5 days and one used 50 mg for 5 days. The best odds ratio was associated with the lower dose (Deaton *et al.* 1990). To date, no specific laboratory test can identify those couples with unexplained infertility who are more likely to respond to clomiphene therapy. The duration of infertility, however, may provide some guidance.

In one randomized trial, the greatest relative increase in conception rates occurred when clomiphene was given to women who had been infertile for more than three years (Glazener *et al*. 1990). A similar finding was observed in a cohort study where the relative likelihood of pregnancy, after adjusting for other prognostic factors, was significantly greater than unity only in those couples who had a duration of infertility greater than 36 months (Collins *et al*. 1991). Thus clomiphene treatment appears to be more valuable in the case of prolonged unexplained fertility. Its benefits are unclear if the infertility is of less than 36 months duration.

Clomiphene is a therapy which has been widely used among women with infertility due to ovulation disorders, and, with more than two decades of experience, its side-effects are reasonably predictable. As an empirical therapy for couples with unexplained fertility, clomiphene offers advantages in dollars and time costs that are not available with many other treatments. Pending confirmation or refutation by further studies, the use of a relatively simple therapy such as clomiphene is clinically justified in such couples. Its use should not be recommended where the duration of infertility is less than 36 months. The reported effect of clomiphene occurred in trials of four to six months' duration. Whether or not there is a continuing effect of clomiphene administration after six months is unknown.

When the medication is used for anovulatory women, the majority of pregnancies which occur do so in the first six months of treatment (Shalev *et al*. 1989). The question of when to discontinue unsuccessful empirical treatments, including clomiphene, is discussed in greater detail in Chapter 16.

Human menopausal gonadotrophins with or without intrauterine insemination

Superovulation with gonadotrophins might improve the pregnancy rate in patients with unexplained infertility simply by exposing a larger number of oocytes to the chance of fertilization. It has also been suggested that unrecognized minor endocrine disturbances in the ovulatory process could be corrected by the use of this treatment.

Intrauterine insemination in natural ovulatory cycles has not been shown to improve fertility. It has seemed reasonable to assume that a combination of superovulation with intrauterine insemination might improve fertility.

Whether treatment with superovulation with gonadotrophins (HMG) alone, or in combination with intrauterine insemination (IUI), improves fertility is a question that has not been addressed in uniformly designed studies. Some make use of HMG only, while others use the combination. Some make use of untreated control groups, and others use either HMG or IUI treatment as a control for the combination. These differences create a heterogeneity among the studies that is further complicated by a dearth of prospective designs. This section will describe two uncontrolled studies and review four comparative studies which to date have addressed the question at least in part.

Uncontrolled studies of the use of HMG with IUI for the treatment of unexplained infertility

In the largest reported study there were 17 pregnancies during 116 cycles of treatment, achieving a fecundity of 0.15, or 15 per cent per cycle (Dodson and Haney 1991). Yovich and Matson (1988) reported on 68 couples with unexplained infertility of 61 months' duration, who received 134 treatment cycles with ovulation stimulation and intrauterine insemination (2 cycles per couple). Twelve (18 per cent) of the women conceived. The reported fecundity was 9 per cent per cycle. It is not possible, however, to identify separately from their data the results for couples who were treated with clomiphene citrate, human menopausal gonadotrophin, or a combination of the two drugs.

Although these two studies suggest that HMG with IUI might hold promise as a treatment for unexplained infertility, the lack of untreated controls does not permit this information to be translated into routine clinical practice.

Comparative studies

Comparative studies with retrospective cross-over designs (Chaffkin *et al.* 1991; Corson *et al.* 1989) which include only a few patients

Table 15.7 *Human menopausal gonadotrophin (HMG) with intrauterine insemination (IUI) in the treatment of unexplained infertility*

Authors	Patients	Number of pregnancies/patients HMG and IUI	Control	Relative likelihood of pregnancy†	Study design
Control Treatment: none or IUI alone					
Daly 1989	67	8/20	20/47	0.9 (0.3,3.0)	Cohort
Serhal *et al*. 1988	30	6/15	1/15	9.3 (0.8,243)	Cohort
Welner *et al*. 1988*	87	3/39	2/48	1.9 (0.3,15.5)	Cohort
Control Treatment: HMG alone					
Crosignani 1991	236	36/158	9/78	2.3 (0.9,5.4)	RCT
Serhal *et al*. 1988	40	6/15	3/25	4.9 (0.8,32.6)	Cohort

* Treatment was HMG alone
† Odds ratio (95 per cent CI)

with unexplained infertility, and studies with diagnostic and treatment stratification together with cross-over from cycle to cycle (Martinez *et al*. 1991), may improve our understanding of some mechanisms that apply, but do not directly address the question 'Is HMG with IUI an effective treatment for unexplained infertility?' Four other clinical studies have included some form of comparison group (Table 15.7).

Welner *et al*. (1988) compared the effect on fertility of HMG alone in a group of 39 women with 48 women who did not receive such therapy. The average duration of infertility in these groups was 83 and 78 months respectively, which may explain the low pregnancy rates, 3 in 39 treated women (8 per cent) versus 2 in 48 untreated women (4 per cent).

Serhal *et al*. (1988) compared IUI alone with HMG alone and with HMG plus IUI. The study groups differed with respect to the duration of their infertility, and the age of the female partner. In this report, HMG alone and IUI alone yielded similar pregnancy rates. The combination of HMG and IUI appeared to be superior to either.

Daly (1989) compared HMG and IUI with no treatment in a group of 67 couples with unexplained infertility, all of whom were shown by ultrasound monitoring to be free of abnormal follicular dynamics. In this selected set of couples, patients were not randomly allocated, but rather elected whether or not to have therapy. The pregnancy rate per 100 treated cycles (4.2 per cent) was not significantly higher than that observed per 100 untreated cycles (3.5 per cent).

A large multi-centre randomized trial was reported by Crosignani *et al.* in September 1990 at the annual meeting of the European Society for Human Reproduction and Embryology in Milan, Italy (Crosignani *et al.* 1991). The design evaluated several treatments, each of which was compared with HMG alone. Because cross-over occurred in the second cycle of the study, only the data from the 444 first cycles are included in this summary. There were 9 pregnancies in 78 HMG-only cycles, 36 in 158 HMG and IUI cycles, 3 in 17 cycles of HMG and intraperitoneal insemination treatment, 37 in 114 GIFT cycles, and 21 in 67 IVF cycles. It would appear from these data that HMG with IUI is superior to HMG alone.

Table 15.7 summarizes the results of the four comparative studies. The odds ratios and 95 per cent confidence intervals have been calculated. HMG alone does not appear to be superior to no treatment (Welner *et al.* 1988). HMG alone was used as the control in two comparisons (Crosignani *et al.* 1991; Serhal *et al.* 1988), and, as it does not appear to be superior to no treatment, it may serve as a surrogate for no treatment, as does IUI alone. In all the studies the 95 per cent confidence intervals overlap unity. Given the variety of active control treatments and the uncertainty about whether such active controls truly are placebos, it seems unjustified to combine the results of these studies. Although it is difficult to avoid suspecting that HMG plus IUI may be an effective treatment for unexplained infertility, this conclusion remains unproven by conventional statistical standards.

In vitro fertilization (IVF) and its variants

In vitro fertilization or some variant of this basic technique is now the last resort in the treatment of almost all infertile patients, and yet to date no studies are available which compare the pregnancy rates in patients with unexplained infertility treated by these methods with the rates in similar untreated patients. In the previous sections of this chapter, a single question was asked: does this treatment improve fertility? While with respect to IVF the literature to date does not address the question satisfactorily, it does provide information about the prognosis for patients treated by these methods. A limited range of studies compare *in vitro* technique (IVF) with gamete intrafallopian transfer (GIFT), and GIFT with HMG plus IUI.

The prognosis for patients with unexplained infertility treated by
in vitro *fertilization*

Lower fertilization rates were initially reported among women with unexplained infertility undergoing IVF, when compared with women who had bilateral tubal obstruction (Mahadevan and Trounson 1984). Table 15.8 summarizes more recent information on this comparison, including the comprehensive date from the United States for 1989, and reports from single centres in France and Australia. Although some differences were observed, the end result in the three reports is that the pregnancy rate per transfer was approximately equivalent in unexplained infertility and tubal infertility.

Comparisons of IVF and GIFT procedures

Two of the series shown in Table 15.8 compare the results of IVF and GIFT. Hartz *et al*. (1991) have reported that the GIFT clinical pregnancy rate (33 per cent) is significantly superior to the IVF clinical pregnancy rate (23 per cent). The proportions with live births (respectively 26 per cent and 20 per cent) were not statistically different. Yovich and Matson (1988) also reported that the pregnancy rate with GIFT was significantly superior. These observations were collected over time (Yovich and Matson 1988) or from different centres (Hartz *et al*. 1991). Whether IVF or GIFT is superior can only be answered conclusively within the framework of a single trial.

Leeton *et al*. (1987) alternately allocated couples with unexplained infertility to treatment with GIFT or IVF. There were 7 pregnancies (19 per cent) among 37 cycles of GIFT and 6 pregnancies (20 per cent) among 30 IVF cycles (Table 15.9). Similarly, there was no significant preference for either treatment in the data from the first cycle of the European study (Crosignani *et al*. 1991).

Table 15.8 *Pregnancy rates in unexplained infertility and tubal infertility with the use of IVF and GIFT*

Authors	Diagnosis	Number of cycles	Pregnancies/transfer (per cent)	
			IVF	GIFT
Hartz *et al.* 1991	Unexplained	1042	58/247 (23 per cent)	126/378 (33 per cent)
	Tubal	3779	468/2348 (20 per cent)	82/335 (24 per cent)
Audibert *et al.* 1989	Unexplained	217	30/121 (25 per cent)	NA
	Tubal	748	146/554 (26 per cent)	NA
Yovich and Matson 1988*	Unexplained	129	8/60 (13 per cent)	20/69 (29 per cent)
	Tubal	624	78/550 (14 per cent)	21/74 (28 per cent)

* Overall pregnancy rate per oocyte collection

Table 15.9 A comparison of pregnancy rates with GIFT and IVF among couples with unexplained infertility

| Authors | Pregnancy/cycle (per cent) | | Relative likelihood of pregnancy with GIFT* |
	IVF	GIFT	
Leeton *et al.* 1984	6/30 (20 per cent)	7/37 (19 per cent)	0.93 (0.24, 3.7)
Crosignani *et al.* 1991	21/77 (27 per cent)	37/114 (32 per cent)	1.28 (0.65, 2.5)

* Odds ratio (95 per cent CI)

Although data from case series seem to suggest that there is a relative advantage of GIFT over IVF, the two studies which have to date evaluated this question with the use of comparative methodology have failed to substantiate this hypothesis. It must be remarked that in both the number of treatments reported was relatively small, and consequently both studies lack the statistical power to exclude a small difference.

Comparisons of GIFT with HMG plus IUI

Kaplan *et al.* (1989) retrospectively compared GIFT with HMG plus IUI among couples with unexplained infertility. Using multiple logistic regression GIFT was 3.3 (95 per cent CI: 1.5, 6.5) better than superovulation with intrauterine insemination.

Two prospective studies have also compared these treatments, a recent within-patient comparison from a single centre in the United Kingdom (Iffland *et al.* 1989) and the European multi-centre study (Crosignani *et al.* 1991). There were differences in the ovulation induction protocols, but this single factor seems unlikely to explain the discordant findings of the two studies (Table 15.10). It is important to note that the British study, although prospective, did not feature random allocation; patients were offered a total of three attempts with each treatment, the initial treatment in each case being superovulation with intrauterine insemination, in order to assess the individual response to superovulation. Thereafter treatments were offered 'on a random basis'. Given that superovulation was the 'selection cycle' in the British study, there may have been bias leading to the rather extreme preference for GIFT. The results after random allocation in the European multi-centre study represent superior evidence, and indicate that there may be a small but insignificant preference for GIFT over superovulation procedures.

Summary

Studies using untreated control groups to establish the efficacy of IVF and its variants in cases of unexplained infertility have not yet been reported. Case series suggest that the results of IVF are similar in unexplained infertility and tubal infertility. The best quality of

Table 15.10 *A comparison of pregnancy rates with human menopausal gonadotrophin and intrauterine insemination or GIFT among couples with unexplained infertility*

Authors	Pregnancy/cycle (per cent)		Relative likelihood of pregnancy with GIFT*
	HMG + IUI	GIFT	
Crosignani *et al.* 1991	36/158 (23 per cent)	37/114 (32 per cent)	1.6 (0.9,2.9)
Iffland *et al.* 1991	1/86 (1 per cent)	13/63 (21 per cent)	22.6 (2.9,476)

* Odds ratio (95 per cent CI)

evidence does not discriminate between IVF or GIFT procedures. GIFT appears to be moderately superior to HMG plus IUI.

The efficacy of treatment

As will be seen in the next chapter, the factors affecting treatment decisions among couples with unexplained infertility include issues other than the efficacy of therapy. On the issue of efficacy, however, only clomiphene therapy has been demonstrated by means of acceptable clinical evidence in the form of randomized trials as a treatment with proven superiority over no therapy. On the basis of the best available evidence, HMG plus IUI has possible but unproven benefit, and no studies exist to demonstrate a benefit for *in vitro* fertilization methodology.

16 The management of unexplained infertility

As the previous chapters have outlined, unexplained infertility is an especially frustrating form of infertility, and given the uncertainty about the efficacy of treatment, the options they face may bewilder the infertile couple. One possible response for their physician is that given by Professor Alexander Hamilton, in his 1792 treatise on the management of female complaints '. . . recourse should always be had to the advice of practitioners of eminence'. At the other extreme lies the 'Cure Guaranteed' approach, a marketing stratagem satirized by Bernard Shaw in *The Doctor's Dilemma* (1923). Somewhere between these options a course of action must be found which will provide for the needs of the couple. To reiterate, these needs include:

- the obvious desire to conceive;
- autonomy;
- accurate answers to their questions;
- emotional support; and
- if conception does not occur, the feeling that all reasonable avenues have been explored.

Those who do not conceive must be able to feel that they have done their utmost, so that finally they can dismount from the treadmill of investigations and unsuccessful therapy. Each couple will require an individual plan.

In many respects, infertility is similar to a chronic disease. The intensity of the disorder may wax or wane; spontaneous remission, in this instance resulting in pregnancy, may occur; there is no guaranteed cure; and those suffering from the condition may educate themselves and become partners in their health care. Given that information is a key element in the individual's or the couple's feelings of control, it is appropriate to consider that knowledge is an essential tool for the couple (Lalos *et al.* 1985). A structured plan is also important, because only through contributing to such a plan and keeping their vision of the plan in mind can the couple express their autonomy. Finally, even in the least autocratic health-care setting, the availability of counselling is an essential safeguard against the emotional pressure associated with infertility and its management.

This chapter will review the components of decision-making in infertility practice, summarize the results of that decision-making as shown by the Canadian experience, review the knowledge that may be required to meet the patient's needs, and lastly provide a framework from which individualized plans may be developed.

DECISION-MAKING

Once the diagnosis of unexplained fertility has been established the couple, acting upon information provided by the physician, must make a series of decisions. In very general terms these involve choices between:

- active treatment or expectancy;
- treatment options if active treatment is chosen;
- continuing or discontinuing an individual treatment; and
- continuing or discontinuing treatment altogether.

The physician must also constantly make decisions, the most important of which is choosing which treatment options to discuss. This section will examine the decision-making process from the perspectives of the theoretical models, the physician, and the patient. It will conclude by discussing the results of decision-making in practice.

Theoretical models

The process of decision-making in clinical practice has been studied from three points of view: decision analysis, decision theory, and the inquiry into how innovation diffuses among clinicians. Decision analysis comprises the study of evidence for the utility of diagnostic and treatment decisions in order to determine the value of practice protocols; such studies make use of clinical outcomes to quantify the effect of a decision at each node in the decision-tree (Clark 1989).

The study of decision theory deals with the components of clinical decision-making. One theoretical model that has been applied in the general area of reproductive medical care postulates that decisions to prescribe are based in part on preformed attitudes and in part on current demands (Ajzen and Fishbein 1980). For the prescriber the preformed attitudes are shaped by education and influential clinical authorities; the current demands include a perception of what peers would do in this circumstance and a conception of what the patient's needs may be. These are interacting with independent preformed attitudes in the patient, and with a set of perceived social pressures bearing on the patient. Much of the support for such models comes from studies of behaviour, and there is little systematized research to indicate to what extent such formally tested models are applicable in clinical practice in infertility.

The third influence on clinical decisions takes into account how changes in practice occur at the local level; the diffusion of innovative ideas and new technology among medical professionals is an area in need of study, although influential clinicians seem to play a role and certain elements of physician learning (age, type of practice, sources of drug information, and number of professional journals read) also contribute to the observed variance in prescribing patterns among physicians (Joyce *et al*. 1968).

Physician factors

The informal scheme shown in Fig. 16.1 puts into perspective the way physicians may approach infertility-treatment decisions. The clinician's experience is important and can have a powerful influence on decision-making. In the management of infertility, even after an effect on fertility has been tested formally, as in the case of bromocriptine therapy, the unproven therapy continues to be prescribed in some practices. Also, personal experience with rare side-effects can have an unwarranted inhibiting effect on future prescribing.

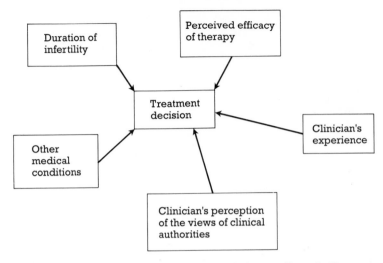

Fig. 16.1 *Factors considered by the physician which may affect infertility treatment decisions.*

Clinicians' perspectives of the views of their peers and the views of respected authorities must also be taken into account.

Patient factors

The perception of patients' attitudes is a further important component of the clinical decision-making process. Women with reproductive problems and couples with infertility in the 1990s are better equipped than ever before to participate in decision-making, a fact which is in part a benefit from the greater public interest in health during the 1980s. This means that, to a greater extent than ever before, clinical decisions can be tailored to the needs of the individual. Feelings about infertility treatment are also influenced by the patient's age, and this is true in particular among women who perceive that they have a limited time in which to conceive. Distance to be travelled, flexibility of daily home and work schedules, and the cost of treatment are relatively simple factors to understand. Less obvious are the differences among patients with respect to attitudes towards decision-making and risk-taking. Some time at least should be taken to evaluate how individual patients view

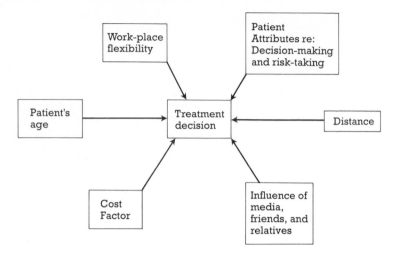

Fig. 16.2 *Patient-related factors that may influence infertility treatment decisions.*

decision-making and risk-taking in general. Finally, the influence of the media, friends, and relatives on the couple's decisions cannot be ignored. These influences are illustrated in Fig. 16.2.

Treatment decision-making in practice

Factors affecting the treatment decision

The CITES report evaluated factors that contributed to a treatment decision among 470 couples attending infertility clinics associated with medical schools in Canada. Of these, 130 couples were selected for treatment, and these couples had a longer mean duration of infertility (48 versus 36 months) and were more likely to have had a laparoscopy as part of the investigation (72 per cent versus 48 per cent). In a logistic regression analysis, however, the independent determinants of treatment were time under observation and laparoscopy status; the duration of infertility was only a minor determinant of treatment. Couples remaining under observation for more than 12 months after registering in an infertility clinic were three times as likely to be treated for their continuing infertility. Thus it is the passage of time after coming to the current source of health care (clinic or physician) that influences treatment, not the total duration of infertility. The age of either partner, the pregnancy history, and whether either partner had received previous treatment did not effect whether treatment was prescribed. In particular, measures of social class, occupational classification, and income did not influence the treatment decision (Collins *et al.* 1991).

Clinical features associated with treatment

How such treatment decisions apply in daily practice is of some interest to clinicians, considering the forces which influence treatment decisions. The tables in this section are based on the same data as those cited above (Collins *et al.* 1991), with the addition of a further 92 couples, 51 of whom were treated. In Table 16.1 clinical information is shown for couples having their first treatment, grouped according to type of treatment. The average duration of infertility for the treated couples was 50 months, and their treatment started on average 7 months after registration, or typically after 57 months of infertility. Patients who had *in vitro* fertilization were older and less likely to have secondary infertility, their duration of infertility was longer, and their family income was higher. As would be expected, raw pregnancy rates among the treated patients were lower than those among the untreated patients, the latter being influenced by pregnancy during the waiting time for treatment.

Table 16.2 shows similar descriptive characteristics of couples undergoing subsequent treatments. One hundred and thirty-nine of the treated cases had only a single treatment, but 42 went on to 2, 3, or 4 regimens. One couple who had the first treatment within two months of registration actually started four more treatments in the next year. Although the trend is not significant, it is notable that the proportion with infrequent intercourse is increasingly higher with repeated treatment, while the pregnancy rates are somewhat lower. Such data underline the hazards that arise from reporting the uncontrolled results of treatment among couples with unexplained infertility.

Table 16.1 *Clinical characteristics and timing of the first treatment decision among couples with unexplained infertility*

First treatment	Number of cases	Duration of infertility (months)	Female age (yrs)	Secondary infertility (per cent)	Coitus < ×2 per wk (per cent)	Income ($000s)	Time to start of first treatment (months)	Proportion pregnant (per cent)
Untreated	381	39	30.0	24.9	15.7	44.8	●	32.3
Clomiphene	110	44	30.6	26.4	17.3	43.9	5.8	19.1
IUI	14	49	32.0	14.3	35.7	43.9	4.6	21.4
IVFGIFT	29	77	32.9	10.3	37.9	68.9	12.9	10.3
Other	28	38	29.4	35.7	3.6	34.1	6.7	21.4
Total	562	42	30.3	24.7	17.1	44.6	7.0	27.8

Data from the Canadian Infertility Therapy Evaluation Study (Vutyavanich and Collins 1991)

Table 16.2 *Clinical characteristics and timing of subsequent treatment decisions among couples with unexplained infertility*

Treatment number	Number of cases	Duration of infertility (months)	Female age (yrs)	Secondary infertility	Coitus < ×2 per wk (per cent)	Income ($000s)	Time to start of first treatment (months)	Proportion pregnant
0	381	39	30.0	24.9	15.7	44.8	●	32.3
1	139	47	30.6	21.6	17.3	43.8	6.9	23.7
2	28	59	31.7	28.6	25.0	44.9	16.5	10.7
3	8	56	33.5	50.0	37.5	42.9	22.9	12.5
4	6	44	29.1	20.0	40.0	●	32.2	0.0
Total	562	42	30.3	24.7	17.1	44.6		28.5

Data from the Canadian Infertility Therapy Evaluation Study (Vuryavanich and Collins 1991)

TOOLS FOR DECISION-MAKING

Rational decisions, inasmuch as any human choices are truly rational, can only be made from a foundation of accurate knowledge. This section will describe a method whereby information about unexplained fertility and its treatment can be shared.

The mythology

One function of the clinician is to dispel the mythology which has arisen around infertility treatment. The mythology is composed of non-expert myths, medical myths, marketing myths, and research myths. All may be well-meaning, but all are capable of exploiting and disturbing couples. The boxer-shorts recommendation was made, for example, to Samuel Pepys in the 1660s before the discovery of sperm by Leeuwenhoek in 1687 (Fraser 1984; Heniger 1973). Prescribing coital patterns, using basal temperatures, and purchasing urine test kits are practices that arise more from mythology than from any evidence of efficacy. The use of written material is often more effective than the spoken word in helping couples to understand why a cherished belief may be incorrect.

Establishing a prognosis

Figure 16.3 is modified from Fig. 12.1, and serves as a good basis for educating couples about their prognosis. This figure illustrates the adjusted probability of pregnancy after a period of infertility. A more individualized prognosis is possible if an adjustment is introduced for the factors present in the individual couple which are known significantly to affect the prognosis (Table 16.3). The pregnancy rate is nearly double, for example, among couples with secondary infertility, and the prognosis is similarly better with less than 36 months' duration of infertility. The female partner's age decreases the fertility of approximately 9 per cent for every year of age beyond 30. Applying arithmetical adjustments in this way is at best an approximation; the predicted pregnancy rate for couples with 1 or 2 years' duration of infertility probably takes into account

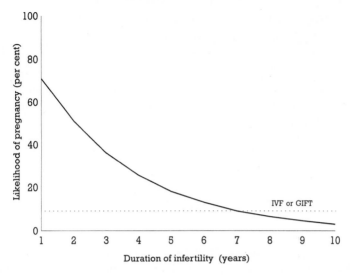

Fig. 16.3 *Duration of infertility and the likelihood of pregnancy (———). IVF or GIFT results United States, 1989: 2104 pregnancies among 17 970 couples (11.7 per cent) (..........) (Hartz et al. 1991).*

such factors as secondary infertility, so that the temptation to double the basic pregnancy rate of 71 per cent must be avoided. Similarly, at the far extreme, the figure of 3 per cent should probably not be reduced by applying negative factors. Within the central portions of the figure, however, which account for the majority of couples considering treatment, it is reasonably accurate for working out a prognosis tailored to the individual couple.

Applying treatment factors to the prognostic model

Although prognosis models are limited by comparison with the reality of clinical and biological variability, they can serve to help us understand the role of treatment (Table 16.4). With more than three years' duration of infertility, for example, the fecundability is doubled in those who use clomiphene for about six months. Treatment with IUI and HMG, separately or together, may offer similar benefits, but these benefits are unproven. IVF and GIFT have not been evaluated in comparison with no treatment in cases of

Table 16.3 *Summary of significant prognostic factors for fertility among untreated couples with unexplained infertility**

Clinical factor	Relative effect
Secondary infertility	2.4 times better
Duration of infertility (mean 39 months)	
for each further month	2 per cent lower
for each further year	26 per cent lower
if less than three years	2.3 times better
Age of the female partner (mean 30 years)	
for each further year	9 per cent lower
if less than 30 years	1.6 times better

* Modified from Table 12.5

unexplained infertility. Registry reports (Table 15.8) indicate the likelihood of pregnancy per cycle may be 1 to 10 times the various rates shown in Table 15.2 for untreated couples (Hartz *et al.* 1991).

How long to treat: treatment as a therapeutic trial

As any treatment for infertility is initiated, an important point should be established: when will this treatment stop? A high proportion of normal couples will conceive within six to nine months, and therefore six to nine months represents a reasonable end-point for infertility therapy. If the therapy has corrected some unknown fertility defect and restored the couple to normal fertility, pregnancy would have been expected in the majority of cases after six to nine months. Continuing the therapy after this time is less likely to be productive.

The duration of the clomiphene trials reported in Chapter 15 was 4 to 6 months; the average duration of therapy in many superovulation programmes is shorter, and probably approaches the mean of 2.2 cycles reported in the largest study (Dodson and Haney 1991). Given the intensity of such treatments it may be unrealistic to expect many couples to continue for even six months.

Regardless of the information drawn on to establish a rational endpoint, discussion about the length of therapy and the decision about when to stop should take place before treatment commences.

Table 16.4 *Relative effect of treatment on fertility among couples with unexplained infertility*

Treatment	Treatment effect relative to no treatment
Clomiphene	2.1 (1.2–3.6)[a]*
IUI	2.1 (0.6–6.9)[b]†
HMG	1.9 (0.3–15.5)[c]‡
HMG + IUI	0.9 to 2.3[d]§
IVF	1 to 10[e]¶

* Typical odds ratio (95 per cent CI) Table 15.6
† Typical odds ratio (95 per cent CI), Martinez *et al.* 1991; Kirby *et al.* 1991
‡ Odds ratio (95 per cent CI), Welner *et al.* 1988
§ Daly 1989 (relative to no treatment); Crosignani *et al.* 1991 (relative to HMG alone)
¶ American Fertility Society registry results (Table 15.8) relative to fecundability among various groups of untreated couples (Table 15.2)

If couples can establish their destination before they begin their journey they are much more likely to recognize when they have arrived.

Understanding the benefits, costs, and risks

The lack of a proven rationale for therapy and the lack of proven effectiveness of many of the treatments suggests that patients' wishes should count heavily in the choice. Although no summary can take into account individual preferences and willingness to take risks, the information shown in Table 16.5 can be adapted to individual clinic practices, and will help patients to understand the costs in money and time and the adverse effects. The adverse effects score is the product of arbitrary assignments, and the lack of published data that could be assembled in such a form is further evidence of the need for better data upon which to base this important decision. In addition to the numerical data shown, details of the procedures, the protocols, and the specific adverse affects may also affect the individual couple's choice.

Table 16.5 *Summary of issues affecting the choice of therapy for couples with unexplained infertility*

Treatment	Cost per cycle ($)*	Time commitment cycle (hrs)	Adverse effect score†
Clomiphene	50	2	1.3
IUI	200	6	1.1
HMG	1200	13	2.0
HMG + IUI	1400	19	2.2
IVF	1500+	24	2.4

* Cost includes drug costs, and for IUI, home monitoring and processing cost. IVF procedure costs, which range in Canada from 0 to $3500, should be added to the IVF figure.
† These are arbitrary assignments.

Education programmes and how they may help

Busy clinicians will wonder how on earth they can provide this vast array of information for couples trying to make decisions. Even those most sensitive to patient autonomy may retreat to rigid protocols, in the face of the time commitment involved in creating a prognosis, explaining the treatment effects, and going through a structured plan. We have had experience in one clinic with an education programme for such couples. It is given for two hours weekly and lasts for three weeks, outside the regular clinic hours. The material taught includes perspectives on infertility from the diagnostic and historical point of view, a range of information about prognosis, and a description of the benefits, costs, and side-effects of the various treatments. Also included are sessions led by counsellors, which deal with the emotional and interpersonal effects of the infertile state. It is too soon to report the measurable value of such an approach, but the comments of the couples are enthusiastic.

DEVELOPING AN INDIVIDUALIZED PLAN OF MANAGEMENT

Many couples will benefit from participating in the development of a plan for the management of their infertility. Such plans will vary in detail, and, although structured, they allow for change as necessary. New directions can be devised at key points during the course of the infertility:

(1) at initial entry;

(2) after initial diagnosis;

(3) at 36 months' duration of infertility

(4) after any treatment has been completed; and

(5) at any time at the couple's request.

The plan for each couple will usually depend on a long-term view of their prognosis. A choice is initially made between active therapy and observation. The benefits and risks of any active intervention can be presented in a way that is consistent with the couple's prognosis.

Some couples will not be able to make such decisions, and will ask for clinical direction. Under such circumstances, it may be wise to suggest that the couple go home and think about the options before a plan is implemented. With respect to some choices, while the autonomy of the couple is important, the responsible physician may wish to limit the couple's requests. Such limitations might be based on the futility of some options, on ethical concerns, or on concerns about the health-care expenditures. Extreme cases, such as the couple undergoing five different treatments within a year, are very likely to undermine the trust normally placed by infertile couples in their clinical advisers.

Application to hypothetical couples

Figure 16.4 shows graphically how a plan might be constructed. John and Jean have infertility of two years' duration. Jean has never been pregnant, and is 29 years of age. They have intercourse two to three times weekly. Their investigation has included semen analysis values which exceed the World Health Organization cutpoints, and presumptive evidence that Jean is ovulating on a regular basis. The hysterosalpingogram performed six months ago and a laparoscopy performed two weeks ago are both reported to be normal. The diagnosis of unexplained fertility is made, and it is decided that no further diagnostic tests are necessary.

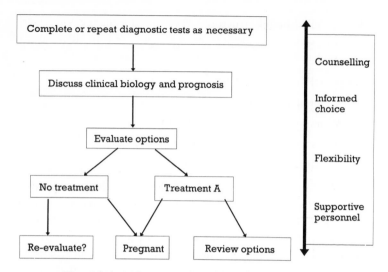

Fig. 16.4 *A clinician's guide to unexplained infertility.*

Figure 16.3 indicates that there is a 51 per cent probability of pregnancy without treatment. The couple's frequency of intercourse does not reduce the prognosis, but Jean's age may improve it by a factor as large as 1.7. In this case, however, because the female partner's age is close to thirty years, it would be preferable to use the yearly age adjustment, which is 0.9 per year of increasing age or 1 ÷ 0.9 per year of decreasing age. For a female partner 29 years of age (1 year below the mean age, 30 years), the likelihood of pregnancy is 51 × 1/0.9, or 56 per cent. After a discussion of the clinical biology of infertility and their prognosis, John and Jean decide to wait a little longer, and they ask for a review in six months.

At the next appointment six months later, because the prognosis remains quite good, they choose to wait a further six months. By that time one year has elapsed since their diagnosis was established, the duration of the infertility is now three years, and Jean is thirty years of age. The probability of pregnancy has fallen to 39 per cent because of the longer duration of infertility (approximately 25 per cent per year, that is 51 × 0.75, or 39 per cent); the age factor is unity at the mean age (30 years). The couple ask about IVF. The success rate in the local clinic is 14 per cent per couple. They will not fall below this expected level for more than a year. As three years of infertility have now elapsed, however, a trial of clomiphene citrate would be indicated, and this is discussed. Their plan will consist of a maximum of six cycles of clomiphene therapy followed by a six-month period without therapy. If by then pregnancy has not occurred they will enrol in the IVF programme for a maximum of three cycles—a course of action which will deplete their financial resources.

An approach based on fecundability may be useful for some couples. For example, a couple with four years' duration of un-explained fertility has completed a clomiphene trial, and they are considering IUI alone while they continue to wait for IVF treatment. Their monthly fecundability is about 2 per cent (Table 12.3, p. 160). Although the best evidence available does not support an IUI effect, it is just possible that a twofold effect might exist (Table 16.4). Thus in a six-month trial the approximate cumulative pregnancy rate might rise from 12 to 24 per cent. Although such effects in part represent bias due to follow-up selection, the side-effects and cost of IUI therapy are reasonably low. What should the couple do? The decision must be theirs.

It would be facile to believe that all cases of unexplained infertility can be worked through so simply. Nevertheless, it is believed that the discussion of such structured, but flexible, patient-driven plans, based upon the best currently available information, is vastly superior to the disorganized 'cure guaranteed' approach described by George Bernard Shaw.

Counselling

From the information provided in Chapter 13 it can easily be predicted that psychosocial disturbances may occur that are not amenable to ordinary clinical management. Couples often feel despair when they hear an honest prognosis. Many couples are despondent after the completion of therapy, especially short-term intensive therapy such as *in vitro* fertilization, without success. Thus couples who are under observation in infertility clinics with or without treatment have a real need for continuing support and counselling.

Couples respond in different ways to continuing childlessness, to the procedures used in infertility investigation and treatment, and to the apparent failure of management when childlessness persists (Mahlstedt 1985). Physicians and other clinical staff can help them to understand the sources of anxiety and stress among infertile couples. Among those with unexplained infertility in particular, uncertainty about the diagnosis and prognosis may aggravate the feelings of one or both partners.

Couples with prolonged infertility frequently change physicians during the course of management, in the hope that any new approach may increase their chances of conception. Changing physicians may also reflect dissatisfaction with the treatment plan, or with the attitude of the physician or other members of the clinical team. Such counselling is provided in many IVF programmes, but many other infertile couples may need access to knowledgeable counselling by social workers, psychologists, or interested psychiatrists. For infertile couples, counselling has more value if the professional involved has a knowledge of the clinical and biological basis of infertility.

SUMMARY

In regard to the efficacy of treatments for unexplained fertility, clinicians often say 'what a good idea, let's try it' rather than 'what a good idea, let's test it'. In regard to the treatment of the individual couple, the former model, which in this case might be expressed as 'let's give this a try', followed after a certain amount of time by the anguished question 'now what?' must be avoided. This chapter has suggested a possible approach to the management of unexplained infertility, an approach which embraces some, but not all, of the ideas developed in the course of this book. Counting heavily in every decision are the needs and wishes of each couple. Also, given the importance of continuing childlessness and the desire for conception on the part of the infertile couple, it is only resonable to point out that their clinicians can help couples immeasurably by sharing their comprehensive knowledge with the couple. Couples who have the knowledge to participate in the development of an individualized plan of management are less likely to be dissatisfied with disappointing results; they rightly share in rewarding results.

References

Abarbanel, A. R. and Bach, G. (1959). Group psychotherapy for the infertile couple. *Int. J. Fertil.*, **4**, 151–60.

Abdel-Latif, A., Mathur, S., Rust, P. F., Fredericks, C. M., Abdel-Aal, H., and Williamson, H. O. (1986). Cytotoxic sperm antibodies inhibit sperm penetration of zona-free hamster eggs. *Fertil. Steril.*, **45**, 542–9.

Abdulla, U., Diver, J., Hipkin, L., and Davis, J. (1983). Plasma progesterone levels as an index of ovulation. *Br. J. Obstet. Gynecol.*, **90**, 543–8.

Abraham, G. E., Maroulis, G. B., and Marshall, J. R. (1974). Evaluation of ovulation and corpus luteum function using measurements of plasma progesterone. *Obstet. Gynecol.*, **44**, 522–5.

Ackerman, S. B., Graff, D., van Uem, J. F. H. M., Swanson, R. J., Veeck, L. L., Acosta, A. A., *et al.* (1984). Immunologic infertility and *in vitro* fertilization. *Fertil. Steril.*, **42**, 474–7.

Adashi, E. Y. (1984). Clomiphene citrate: mechanism(s) and site(s) of action—a hypothesis revisited. *Fertil. Steril.*, **42**, 331–44.

Adeghe, J.-H., Cohen, J., and Sawers, S. R. (1986). Relationship between local and systemic autoantibodies to sperm, and evaluation of immunobead test for sperm surface antibodies. *Acta Eur. Fertil.*, **17**, 99–105.

Aedo, A. R., Landgren, B. M., Cekan, Z., and Diczfalusy, E. (1976). Studies on the pattern of circulating steroids in the normal menstrual cycle. *Acta Endocrinol.*, **82**, 600–16.

Ahlgren, M. (1975). Sperm transport to and survival in the human fallopian tube. *Gynecol. Invest.*, **6**, 206–14.

Aitken, R. J. J. (1983). The zona-free hamster egg penetration test. In *Male infertility* (ed. T. B. Hargreave), pp. 75–86. Springer-Verlag, Berlin.

Aitken, R. J., Best, F. S. M., Warner, P., and Templeton, A. (1984). A prospective study of the relationship between semen quality and fertility in cases of unexplained infertility. *J. Androl.*, **5**, 297–303.

Ajzen, I. and Fishbein, M. (1980). *Understanding attitudes and predicting social behaviour*, p. 22. Prentice-Hall, Englewood Cliffs, NJ.

Albrecht, B. H., Fernando, R. S., Regas, J., and Betz, G. (1985). A new method for predicting and confirming ovulation. *Fertil. Steril.*, **44**, 200–5.

Alexander, N. J. (1981). Evaluation of male infertility with an *in vitro* cervical mucus penetration test. *Fertil. Steril.*, **36**, 201–8 (Abstract).

Alexander, N. J. (1984). Antibodies to human spermatozoa impede sperm penetration of cervical mucus or hamster eggs. *Fertil. Steril.*, **41**, 433–9.

Alexander, N. J. and Anderson, D. J. (1979). Vasectomy: consequences of autoimmunity to sperm antigens. *Fertil. Steril.*, **32**, 253–60.

Alexander, N. J. and Anderson, D. J. (1987). Immunology of semen. *Fertil. Steril.*, **47**, 192–205.

Alexander, N. J. and Bearwood, D. (1984). An immunosorption assay for antibodies to spermatozoa: comparison with agglutination and immunobilization tests. *Fertil. Steril.*, **41**, 270–6.

Allen, E., Pratt, J. P., Newell, Q. U., and Bland, L. (1928). Recovery of human ova from the uterine tubes: time of ovulation in the menstrual cycle. *JAMA*, **91**, 1018–20.

Alper, M. and Siebel, M. M. (1986). Aberrant surge of luteinizing hormone in women with endometriosis (unpublished MS).

Alper, M. M., Garner, P. R., Spence, J. E. H., and Quarrington, A. M. (1986). Pregnancy rates after hysterosalpingography with oil- and water-soluble contrast media. *Obstet. Gynecol.*, **68**, 6–9.

Amann, R. P. (1979). Computerized measurements of sperm velocity and percentage of motile sperm. In *The spermatozoon* (ed. D. W. Fawcett and J. M. Bedford), pp. 431–5. Urban and Schwarzenberg, Baltimore.

American Fertility Society (1985). Revised American Fertility Society Classification of Endometriosis. *Fertil. Steril.*, **43**, 351–2.

American Fertility Society (1986). *Investigation of the infertile couple*, pp. 25–7. American Fertility Society, Birmingham, Alabama.

Anderson, D. J. and Hill, J. A. (1988). Cell-mediated immunity in infertility. *Am. J. Reprod. Immunol. Microbiol.*, **17**, 22–30.

Anderson, D. J., Bach, D. L., Yunis, E. J., and DeWolf, W. C. (1982). Major histocompatibility antigens are not expressed on human epididymal sperm. *J. Immunol.*, **129**, 452–4.

Andrews, W. C. (1979). Luteal phase defects. *Fertil. Steril.*, **32**, 501–9.

Annos, T., Thompson, I. E., and Taymor, M. L. (1980). Luteal phase deficiency and infertility: difficulties encountered in diagnosis and treatment. *Obstet. Gynecol.*, **55**, 705–10.

Ansbacher, R., Keung-Yeung, K., and Behrman, S. J. (1973). Clinical significance of sperm antibodies in infertile couples. *Fertil. Steril.*, **24**, 305–8.

Aral, S. O. and Cates jun. W. (1983). The increasing concern with infertility: why now? *JAMA*, **250**, 2327–31.

Asch, R. H. (1976). Laparoscopic recovery of sperm from peritoneal fluid in patients with negative or poor Sims–Huhner test. *Fertil. Steril.*, **27**, 1111–14.

Asch, R. H., Balmaceda, J. P., Ellsworth, L. R., and Wong, P. C. (1986). Preliminary experiences with gamete intrafallopian transfer (GIFT). *Fertil. Steril.*, **45**, 366–71.

Asherman, J. G. (1948). Amenorrhoea traumatica (atretica). *J. Obstet. Gynecol. Br. Emp.*, **55**, 23–30.

Audibert, F., Hedon, B., Arnal, F., Humeau, C., Badoc, E., Virenque, V., *et al.* (1989). Results of IVF attempts in patients with unexplained infertility. *Hum. Reprod.*, **4**, 766–71.

Auletta, F. J. and Flint, A. P. F. (1988). Mechanisms controlling corpus luteum function in sheep, cows, non-human primates, and women, especially in relation to the time of luteolysis. *Endocrin. Rev.*, **9**, 88–105.

Ausmanas, M., Tureck, R. W., Ben-Rafael, Z., Lopez, I., Mastroianni, L., and Blasco, L. (1986). Immunologic infertility and *in vitro* fertilization (IVF). *Fertil. Steril.*, **46**, 107–(Abs. 309 Prog. Suppl.).

Austin, C. R. (1951). Observations of the penetration of the sperm into the mammalian egg. *Aust. J. Sci. Res.*, **(B)4**, 581–96.

Austin, C. R. (1975). Membrane fusion events in fertilization. *J. Reprod. Fertil.*, **44**, 155–66.

Ayvaliotis, B., Bronson, R., Rosenfeld, D., and Cooper, G. (1985). Conception rates in couples where autoimmunity to sperm is detected. *Fertil. Steril.*, **43**, 739–42.

Badawy, S. Z. A., Marshall, L., Gabal, A. A., and Nusbaum, M. L. (1982). The concentration of 13,14-dihydro-15-keto prostaglandin F2-alpha and prostaglandin E2 in peritoneal fluid of infertile patients with and without endometriosis. *Fertil. Steril.*, **38**, 166–70.

Badawy, S. Z. A., Cuenca, V., Stitzel, A., Jacobs, R. D. B., and Tomar, R. H. (1984*a*). Autoimmune phenomena in infertile patients with endometriosis. *Obstet. Gynecol.*, **63**, 271–5.

Badawy, S. Z. A., El Shaykh, M., Shulman, S., and Cittadino, R. (1984*b*). Circulating sperm antibodies: indications for testing in infertile couples. *Int. J. Fertil.*, **29**, 159–63.

Bain J. and Keene, E. J. (1975). Further evidence for inhibin: changes in serum luteinizing hormone and follicle-stimulating hormone levels after X-irradiation of rat testes. *J. Endocrinol.*, **66**, 279–80.

Baker, T. G. (1981). Oogenesis and ovulation. In *Reproduction in Mammals:*

Book 1. Germ cells and fertilization (ed. C. R. Austin and R. V. Short), pp. 17–45. Cambridge University Press.

Baker, H. W., Clarke, G. N., Hudson, B., McBain, J. C., McGowan, M. P., and Pepperell, R. J. (1983). Treatment of sperm autoimmunity in men. *Clin. Reprod. Fertil.*, **2**, 55–71.

Baker, H. W. G., Burger, H. G., de Kretser, D. M., Hudson, B., Rennie, G. C., and Straffon, W. G. E. (1985). Testicular vein ligation and fertility in men with variococeles. *Br. Med. J.*, **291**, 1678–80.

Balasch, J. and Vanrell, J. A. (1987). Corpus luteum insufficiency and fertility: a matter of controversy. *Hum. Reprod.*, **2**, 557–67.

Balasch, J., Vanrell, J. A., Creus, M., Marquez, M., and Gonzalez-Merlo, J. (1985). The endometrial biopsy for diagnosis of luteal phase deficiency. *Fertil. Steril.*, **44**, 699–701.

Balasch, J., Creus, M., Marquez, M., Burzaco, I., and Vanrell, J. A. (1986). The significance of luteal phase deficiency on fertility: a diagnostic and therapeutic approach. *Hum. Reprod.*, **1**, 145–7.

Barbieri, R. L. (1986). Ca-125 in patients with endometriosis. *Fertil. Steril.*, **45**, 767–9.

Barnea, E. R., Holford, T. R., and McInnes, D. R. A. (1985). Long-term prognosis of infertile couples with normal basic investigations: a life-table analysis. *Obstet. Gynecol.*, **66**, 24–6.

Barratt, C. L. R., Cooke, S., Chauhan, M., and Cooke, I. D. (1989*a*). A prospective randomized controlled trial comparing urinary luteinizing hormone dipsticks and basal body temperature charts with time donor insemination. *Fertil. Steril.*, **52**, 394–7.

Barratt, C, L. R., Havelock, L. M., Harrison, P. E., and Cooke, I. D. (1989*b*). Antisperm antibodies are more prevalent in men with low sperm motility. *Int. J. Androl.*, **12**, 110–16.

Bayer, S. R., Seibel, M. M., Saffan, D. S., Berger, M. J., and Taymor, M. L. (1988). Efficacy of danazol treatment for minimal endometriosis in infertile women: a prospective randomized study. *J. Reprod. Med.*, **33**, 179–83.

Bedford, J. M. (1981). Fertilization. In *Reproduction in mammals: Book 1. Germ cells and fertilization*, 2nd edn (ed. C. R. Austin and R. V. Short), pp. 128–63. Cambridge University Press.

Ben-Jonathan, N. (1985). Dopamine: a prolactin-inhibiting hormone. *Endocrin. Rev.*, **6**, 564–89.

Berger, D. M. (1980). Impotence following the discovery of azoospermia. *Fertil. Steril.*, **34**, 154–6.

Berkowitz, R. S., Alexander, N. J., Goldstein, D. P., and Anderson, D. J. (1985). Reactivity of anti-human sperm monoclonal antibodies with normal placenta, hydatidiform mole, and gestational choriocarcinoma. *Gynecol. Oncol.*, **22**, 334–40.

Bissett, D. L. (1980). Development of a model of human cervical mucus. *Fertil. Steril.*, **33**, 211–12 (Abstract).

Blandau, R. J. (1969). Gamete transport—comparative aspects. In *The mammalian oviduct* (ed. E. S. E. Hafez and R. J. Blandau), pp. 129–62. University of Chicago Press.

Blandau, R. J. (1978). Mechanism of tubal transport—comparative aspects. In *Reversibility of female sterilization*, (ed. I. Brosens and R. Winston), pp. 1–20. Academic Press, London.

Blandau, R. J., Bourdage, R. J., and Halbert, S. A. (1979). Tubal transport. In *The biology of the fluids in the female genital tract* (ed. F. K. Beller and G. F. B. Schumacher), pp. 319–33. Elsevier, Amsterdam.

Blumenfeld, Z., Gershon, H., Makler, A., Stoler, J., and Brandes, J. M. (1986). Detection of antisperm antibodies: a cytotoxicity immobilization test. *Int. J. Fertil.*, **31**, 207–12.

Bornman, M. S., Du Toit, D., Otto, B., Muller, I. I., Hurter, P., and Du Plessis, D. J. (1989). Seminal carnitine, epididymal function and spermatozoal motility. *S. Afr. Med. J.*, **75**, 20–1.

Borth, R., Lunenfeld, B., and deWatteville, H. (1954). Activite gonadotrope d'un extrait d'urines de femmes en menopause. *Experientia*, **10**, 266–9.

Bostofte, E. (1987). Prognostic parameters in predicting pregnancy. *Acta Obstet. Gynecol. Scand.*, **66**, 617–24.

Bostofte, E., Serup, J., and Rebbe, H. (1982). Relation between sperm count and semen volume, and pregnancies obtained during a twenty-year follow-up period. *Int. J. Androl.*, **5**, 267–75.

Bostofte, E., Serup, J., and Rebbe, H. (1984). Relation between number of immobile spermatozoa and fertility. *Andrologia*, **16**, 136–40.

Bostofte, E., Serup, J., and Rebbe, H. (1985). The clinical value of morphological rating of human spermatozoa. *Int. J. Fertil.*, **30**(3), 31–7.

Bostofte, E., Bagger, P., Michael, A., and Stakemann, G. (1990). Fertility prognosis for infertile men: results of follow-up study of semen analysis in infertile men from two different populations evaluated by the Cox regression model. *Fertil. Steril.*, **54**, 1100–6.

Bousquet, D., St. Jacques, S., Roberts, K. D., Chapdelaine, A., and Bleau, G. (1982). Zona pellucida antibodies in a group of women with idiopathic infertility. *Am. J. Reprod. Immunol.*, **2**, 73–8.

Brandt, H., Acott, T. S., Johnson, D. J., and Hoskins, D. D. (1978).

Evidence for an epididymal origin of bovine sperm forward motility protein. *Biol. Reprod.*, 19, 830–5.

Breslow, N. E. and Day, N. E. (1980). Combination of results from a series of 2 × 2 tables; control of confounding. In *Statistical Methods in Cancer Research: Volume 1—The analysis of case–control studies*, 32nd edn (ed. W. Davis), pp. 136–57. IARC Scientific Publications, Lyons.

Bresnick, E. and Taymor, M. L. (1979). The role of counseling in infertility. *Fertil. Steril.*, 32, 154–6.

Bronson, R. A. (1990). Immunology. In *Infertility, a comprehensive text* (ed. M. M. Siebel), pp. 217–34. Appleton and Lange, Norwalk, Connecticut.

Bronson, R. A., Cooper, G. W., and Rosenfeld, D. L. (1981). Membrane-bound sperm-specific antibodies: their role in infertility. In *Bioregulators of reproduction* (ed. H. Vogel and G. Jagiello), pp. 521–7. Academic Press, New York.

Bronson, R. A., Cooper, G. W., and Rosenfeld, D. L. (1982). Sperm-specific isoantibodies and autoantibodies inhibit the binding of human sperm to the human zona pellucida. *Fertil. Steril.*, 38, 724–9.

Bronson, R., Cooper, G., and Rosenfeld, D. (1984). Sperm antibodies: their role in infertility. *Fertil. Steril.*, 42, 171–83.

Bronson, R., Cooper, G., Hjort, T., Ing, R., Jones, W. R., Wang, S. X., *et al.* (1985). Anti-sperm antibodies, detected by agglutination, immobilization, microcytotoxicity and immunobead-binding assays. *J. Reprod. Immun.*, 8, 279–99.

Brooks, J. H., Mortimer, D., and Taylor, P. J. (1988). Failure of hysteroscopic insemination of the fallopian tube in synchronized cycles. *Int. J. Fertil.*, 33, 353–61.

Brosens, I. A. and Vasquez, G. (1976). Fimbrial microbiopsy. *J. Reprod. Med.*, 16, 171–8.

Busolo, F. and Zanchetta, R. (1985). The effect of *Mycoplasma hominis* and *Ureaplasma urealyticum* on hamster egg *in vitro* penetration by human spermatozoa. *Fertil. Steril.*, 43, 110–14.

Buttram, V. C. J. and Reiter, R. C. (1981). Uterine leiomyomata: etiology, symptomatology, and management. *Fertil. Steril.*, 36, 433–45.

Buvat, J., Marcolin, G., Herbaut, J. C., Dehaene, J. L., Verbecq, P., and Fourlinnie, J. C. (1988). A randomized trial of human chorionic gonadotropin support following *in vitro* fertilization and embryo transfer. *Fertil. Steril.*, 49, 458–61.

Calamera, J. C., Brug, O. S., and Vilar, O. (1982). Relation between motility and adenosine triphosphate (ATP) in human spermatozoa. *Andrologia*, 14, 239–41.

Chaffkin, L. M., Nulsen, J. C., Luciano, A. A., and Metzger, D. A. (1991). A comparative analysis of the cycle fecundity rates associated with combined human menopausal gonadotropin (hMG) and intrauterine insemination (IUI) versus either hMG or IUI alone. *Fertil. Steril.*, **55**, 252–7.

Chan, A. K. and Collins, J. A. Steroid hormone treatment of endometriosis-associated infertility: an overview. *Int. Fertil.* (In press.)

Chang, M. C. (1951). Fertilizing capacity of spermatozoa deposited in the fallopian tubes. *Nature*, **168**, 697–8.

Chappel, S. C., Resko, J. A., Norman, R. L., and Spies, H. G. (1981). Studies in Rhesus monkeys on the site where estrogen inhibits gonadotropins: delivery of 17 Beta-estradiols to the hypothalamus and pituitary gland. *J. Clin. Endocrinol. Metab.*, **52**, 1–8.

Check, J. H., Chase, J. S., Nowroozi, K., Wu, C. H., and Adelson, H. G. (1989). Empirical therapy of the male with clomiphene in couples with unexplained infertility. *Int. J. Fertil.*, **34**, 120–2.

Cheesman, K. L., Ben-Nun, I., Chatterton, R. T., and Cohen, M. R. (1982). Relationship of luteinizing hormone, pregnanediol-3-glucuronide, and estriol-16-glucoronide in urine of infertile women with endometriosis. *Fertil. Steril.*, **38**, 542–8.

Chen, C. and Jones, W. R. (1981). Application of a sperm micro-immobilization test to cervical mucus in the investigation of immunologic infertility. *Fertil. Steril.*, **35**, 542–5.

Chikazawa, K., Araki, S., and Tamada, T. (1986). Morphological and endocrinological studies on follicular development during the human menstrual cycle. *J. Clin. Endocrinol. Metab.*, **62**, 305–13.

Chodirker, W. B. and Tomasi, T. B. J. (1963). Gammaglobulin: quantitative relationships in human serum and non-vascular fluids. *Science*, **142**, 1080–1.

Cimino, C., Barba, G., Pellegrini, S., and Perino, A. (1986). Evaluation of sperm immobilizing and sperm agglutinating seric activity in male subjects with or without positive IgG MAR-test belonging to sub-fertile couples with negative or doubtful PCT. *Acta Eur. Fertil.*, **17**, 259–66.

Clark, J. R. (1989). Decision making in surgical practice. *World J. Surg.*, **13**, 245–51.

Clarke, G. N., Stojanoff, A., Cauchi, M. N., McBain, J. C., Speirs, A. L., and Johnston, W. I. H. (1984). Detection of antispermatozoal antibodies of IgA class in cervical mucus. *Am. J. Reprod. Immunol.*, **5**, 61–5.

Clarke, G. N., Elliott, P. G., and Smaila, C. (1985*a*). Detection of sperm antibodies in semen using the immunobead test: a survey of 813 consecutive patients. *Am. J. Reprod. Immunol. Microbiol.*, **7**, 118–23.

Clarke, G. N., Stojanoff, A., Cauchi, M. N., and Johnston, W. I. H. (1985*b*). The immunoglobulin class of antispermatozoal antibodies in serum. *Am. J. Reprod. Immunol. Microbiol.*, **7**, 143–7.

Clarke, G. N., Lopata, A., and Johnston, W. I. H. (1986). Effect of sperm antibodies in females on human *in vitro* fertilization. *Fertil. Steril.*, **46**, 435–41.

Claton, R. N., Channabasavaiah, K., Stewart, J. M., and Catt, K. J. (1982). Hypothalamic regulation of pituitary gonadotropin-releasing hormone receptors: effects of hypothalamic lesions and a gonadotropin-releasing hormone antagonist. *Endocrinol.*, **110**, 1108–15.

Collins, J. A. (1987). Diagnostic assessment of the infertile male partner. *Curr. Prob. Obstet. Gynecol. Infert.*, **10**, 173–224.

Collins, J. A. (1988). Diagnostic assessment of the infertile female partner. *Curr. Prob. Obstet. Gynecol. Fertil.*, **9**, 1–42.

Collins, J. A. (1989*a*). Male infertility: the interpretation of the diagnostic assessment. In *The yearbook of infertility* (ed. D. R. Mishell, C. A. Paulsen, and R. A. Lobo), pp. 45–74. Yearbook Medical Publishers, Chicago.

Collins, J. A. (1989*b*). Natural course of unexplained infertility. In *Proceedings of the Serono Symposium on Unexplained Infertility: Basic and Clinical Aspects*, pp. 71–85. Serono Aries Publishers, Rome.

Collins, J. A. (1990*b*). Superovulation in the treatment of unexplained infertility. *Semin. in Reprod. Endocrin.*, **8**, 165–73.

Collins, J. A. (1990*a*). Diagnostic assessment of the ovulatory process. *Semin. in Reprod. Endocrin.*, **8**, 145–55.

Collins, J. A. and Rowe, T. C. (1989). Age of the female partner is a prognostic factor in prolonged unexplained infertility: a multicentre study. *Fertil. Steril.*, **52**, 15–20.

Collins, J. A., Wrixon, W., Janes, L. B., and Wilson, E. H. (1983). Treatment-independent pregnancy among infertile couples. *New Engl. J. Med.*, **309**, 1201–6.

Collins, J. A., Ying, S., Wilson, E. H., Wrixon, W., and Casper, R. F. (1984). The postcoital test as a predictor of pregnancy among 355 infertile couples. *Fertil. Steril.*, **41**, 703–8.

Collins, J. A., Rand, C. A., Wilson, E. H., Wrixon, W., and Casper, R. F. (1986). The better prognosis in secondary infertility is associated with a higher proportion of ovulation disorders. *Fertil. Steril.*, **45**, 611–16.

Collins, J. A., Milner, R. A., and Rowe, T. C. (1991). The effect of treatment on pregnancy among couples with unexplained infertility. *Int. J. Fertil.*, **36**, 140–52.

Comhaire, F., Vermeulen, L., Ghedira, K., Mas, J., Irvine, S., and Callipolitis, G. (1983). Adenosine triphosphate in human semen: a quantitative estimate of fertilizing potential. *Fertil. Steril.*, 40, 500–4 (Abstract).

Conway, D. I., Glazener, C. M. A., Kelly, N., and Hull, M. G. R. (1985). Routine measurement of thyroid hormones and FSH in infertility not worthwhile. *Lancet*, i, 977–8.

Corenblum, B. and Taylor, P. J. (1981). Mechanisms of control of prolactin release in response to apprehension stress and anaesthesia–surgery stress. *Fertil. Steril.*, 36, 712–15.

Corenblum, B. and Taylor, P. J. (1987). Clomiphene citrate: a diagnostic and therapeutic agent. *Curr. Prob. Obstet. Gynecol. Fertil.*, 10, 287–326.

Corsan, G. H., Ghazi, D., and Kemmann, E. (1990). Home urinary luteinizing hormone immunoassays: clinical applications. *Fertil. Steril.*, 53, 591–601.

Corson, S. L., Batzer, F. R., Marmar, J., and Maislin, G. (1988). The human sperm–hamster egg penetration assay: prognostic value. *Fertil. Steril.*, 49, 328–34.

Corson, S. L., Batzer, F. R., Gocial, B., and Maislin, G. (1989). Intrauterine insemination and ovulation stimulation as treatment of infertility. *J. Reprod. Med.*, 34, 397–406.

Coutts, J. R. T., Adam, A. H., and Fleming, R. (1982). The deficient luteal phase may represent an anovulatory cycle. *Clin. Endocrin.*, 17, 389–94.

Cox, D. R. (1972). Regression models and life tables. *J. R. Stat. Soc. B*, 34, 187–220.

Crosby, I. M. and Moor, R. M. (1984). *Oocyte maturation in* in vitro *fertilization and embryo transfer*, pp. 19–31. Churchill Livingstone, Edinburgh.

Crosby, I. M., Osborn, J. C., and Moor, R. M. (1982). Follicle cell regulation of protein synthesis and developmental competence in sheep oocytes. *J. Reprod. Fertil.*, 62, 575–82.

Crosignani, P. G., Ragni, G., Lombroso, G. C., Scarduelli, C., De Lauretis, L., Cacamo, A., *et al.* (1988). Ovarian stimulation of IVF patients: effects of the reversible hypogonadotrophic state induced by GnRH agonist. *Hum. Reprod.*, 3 (Suppl 2), 39–41.

Crosignani, G., Walters, D. E., and Soliani, A. (1991). The ESHRE multicentre trial on the treatment of unexplained infertility: a preliminary report. *Hum. Reprod.*, 6, 953–8.

Cross, N. L. and Overstreet, J. W. (1987). Glycoconjugates of the human sperm surface: distribution and alterations that accompany capacitation *in vitro*. *Gamete Res.*, 16, 23–35.

Croxatto, H. B. and Ortiz, M. E. S. (1975). Egg transport in the fallopian tube. *Gynecol. Invest.*, **6**, 215–25.

Croxatto, H. B., Ortiz, M. E., Diaz, S., Hess, R., Balmaceda, J., and Croxatto, H.-D. (1978). Studies on the duration of egg transport by the human oviduct: II. Ovum location at various intervals following luteinizing hormone peak. *Am. J. Obstet. Gynecol.*, **132**, 629–34.

Croxatto, H. B., Ortiz, M. E., Diaz, S., and Hess, R. (1979). Attempts to modify ovum transport in women. *J. Reprod. Fertil.*, **55**, 231–7.

Csapo, A. I., Pulkkinen, M. O., Ruttner, B., Sauvage, J. P., and Wiest, W. G. (1972). The significance of the human corpus luteum in pregnancy maintenance. I. Preliminary studies. *Am. J. Obstet. Gynecol.*, **112**, 1061–7.

Cummings, D. C. and Taylor, P. J. (1979). Historical predictability of abnormal laparoscopic findings in the infertile woman. *J. Reprod. Med.*, **23**, 295–8.

Daly, D. C. (1989). Treatment validation of ultrasound-defined abnormal follicular dynamics as a cause of infertility. *Fertil. Steril.*, **51**, 51–7.

Daniluk, J. C. (1988). Infertility: intrapersonal and interpersonal impact. *Fertil. Steril.*, **49**, 982–90.

David, M. P., Ben-Zwi, D., and Langer, L. (1981). Tubal intramural polyps and their relationship to infertility. *Fertil. Steril.*, **35**, 526–31.

Davis, O. K., Berkeley, A. S., Naus, G. J., Cholst, I. N., and Freedman, K. S. (1989). The incidence of luteal phase defect in normal, fertile women, determined by serial endometrial biopsies. *Fertil. Steril.*, **51**, 582–6.

Dawood, M. Y., Khan-Dawood, F. S., and Wilson, jun., L. (1984). Peritoneal fluid prostaglandins and prostanoids in women with endometriosis, chronic pelvic inflammatory disease, and pelvic pain. *Am. J. Obstet. Gynecol.*, **148**, 391–5 (Abstract).

Deaton, J. L., Gibson, M., Blackmer, K. M., Nakajima, S. T., Badger, G. J., and Brumsted, J. R. (1990). A randomized, controlled trial of clomiphene citrate and intrauterine insemination in couples with unexplained infertility or surgically corrected endometriosis. *Fertil. Steril.*, **54**, 1083–8.

DeCherney, A. H., Kort, H., Barney, J. B., and DeVore, G. R. (1980). Increased pregnancy rate with oil-souble hysterosalpingography dye. *Fertil. Steril.*, **33**, 407–10.

De Jong, F. H. and Sharpe, R. M. (1976). Evidence for inhibin-like activity in bovine follicular fluid. *Nature*, **263**, 71–2.

DeVane, G. W. and Guzick, D. S. (1986). Bromocriptine therapy in normoprolactinemic women with unexplained infertility and galactorrhea. *Fertil. Steril.*, **46**, 1026–31.

Dienes, L. and Edsall, G. (1937). Observations on the L-organism of Klieneberger. *Proc. Soc. Exp. Biol. Med.*, **36**, 740–4.

Dmowski, W. P., Radwanska, E., Binor, Z., and Tummon, I. (1988). Immunological aspects of endometriosis. In *Recent advances in the management of endometriosis* (ed. J. A. Rock and K. W. Schweppe), pp. 31–9. Parthenon Publishing Group, Carnforth, Lancs.

Dodson, W. C. and Haney, A. F. (1991). Controlled ovarian hyperstimulation and intrauterine insemination for treatment of infertility. *Fertil. Steril.*, **55**, 457–67.

Dodson, W. C., Whitesides, D. B., Hughes, jun., C. L., Easley, H. A., and Haney, A. F. (1987). Superovulation with intrauterine insemination in the treatment of infertility: a possible alternative to gamete intrafallopian transfer and in vitro fertilization. *Fertil. Steril.*, **48**, 441–5.

Domar, A. D., Seibel, M. M., and Benson, H. (1990). The mind/body program for infertility: a new behavioral treatment approach for women with infertility. *Fertil. Steril.*, **53**, 246–9.

Dor, J., Homburg, R., and Rabau, E. (1977). An evaluation of etiologic factors and therapy in 665 infertile couples. *Fertil. Steril.*, **28**, 718–22.

Dorrington, J. H., Vernon, R. G., and Fritz, I. B. (1972). The effects of gonadotrophins on the $3',5'$-AMP levels of seminiferous tubules. *Biochem. Biophys. Res. Commun.*, **46**, 1523–8.

Drake, T. S. and Grunert, G. (1979). A cyclic pattern of sexual dysfunction in the infertility investigation. *Fertil. Steril.*, **32**, 542–5.

Drake, T. S., O'Brien, W. F., Ramwell, P. W., and Metz, S. A. (1981). Peritoneal fluid from thromboxane B2 and 6-keto-prostaglandin F1 alpha in endometriosis. *Am. J. Obstet. Gynecol.*, **140**, 401–4.

Driessen, F., Holwerda, P., Putte, S., and Kremer, J. (1980). The significance of dating an endometrial biopsy for the prognosis of the infertile couple. *Int. J. Fertil.*, **25**, 112–16.

Dubin, L. and Amelar, R. D. (1971). Etiologic factors in 1294 consecutive cases of male infertility. *Fertil. Steril.*, **22**, 469–74.

Duignan, N. M., Jordan, J. A., Coughlan, B., and Logan-Edwards, R. (1972). One thousand consecutive cases of diagnostic laparoscopy. *J. Obstet. Gynecol. Br. Common.*, **79**, 1016–24.

Duncan, J. Matthews (1883). The Gulstonian lectures on the sterility of women. Lecture III, Part I.—Its prevention and cure. *Br. Med. J.*, **1**, 701–3.

Dunphy, B. C., Kay, R., Barratt, C. L. R., and Cooke, I. D. (1989*a*). Is routine examination of the male partner of any prognostic value in the routine assessment of couples who complain of involuntary infertility? *Fertil. Steril.*, **52**, 454–6.

Dunphy, B. C., Neal, L. M., and Cooke, I. D. (1989*b*). The clinical value of conventional semen analysis. *Fertil. Steril.*, **51**, 324–9.

Edwards, R. G. (1980). Fertilization. In *Conception in the human female* (ed. R. G. Edwards), pp. 677–85. Academic Press, London.

Edwards, R. G., Bavister, B. D., and Steptoe, P. C. (1969). Early stages of fertilization *in vitro* of human oocytes matured *in vitro*. *Nature*, **221**, 632–5.

Eggert-Kruse, W., Christmann, M., Gerhard, I., Pohl, S., Klinga, K., and Runnebaum, B. (1989*a*). Circulating antisperm antibodies and fertility prognosis: a prospective study. *Hum. Reprod.*, **4**, 513–20.

Eggert-Kruse, W., Leinhos, G., Gerhard, I., Tilgen, W., and Runnebaum, B. (1989*a*). Prognostic value of *in vitro* sperm penetration into hormonally standardized human cervical mucus. *Fertil. Steril.*, **51**, 317–23.

Eggert-Kruse, W., Gerhard, I., Naher, H., Tilgen, W., and Runnebaum, B. (1990). Chlamydial infection—a female and/or male infertility factor? *Fertil. Steril.*, **53**, 1037–43.

El-minawi, M. F., Abdel-hadi, M., Ibrahim, A. A., and Wahby, O. (1978). Comparative evaluation of laparoscopy and hysterosalpingography in infertile patients. *Obstet. Gynecol.*, **51**, 29–32.

Elkind-Hirsch, K., Goldzieher, J. W., Gibbons, W. E., and Besch, P. K. (1986). Evaluation of the OvuSTICK urinary luteinizing hormone kit in normal and stimulated menstrual cycles. *Obstet. Gynecol.*, **67**, 450–3.

Erickson, G. F., Magoffin, D. A., Dyer, C. A., and Hofeditz, C. (1985). The ovarian androgen-producing cells: a review of structure/ function relationships. *Endocrin. Rev.*, **6**, 371–99.

Everett, J. W. (1969). Neuroendocrine aspects of mammalian reproduction. *Annu. Rev. Physiol.*, **31**, 383–416.

Farrer-Meschan, R. (1971). Importance of marriage counseling to infertility investigation. *Obstet. Gynecol.*, **38**, 316–25.

Fayez, J., Mutie, G., and Schneider, P. (1987). The diagnostic value of hysterosalpingography and hysteroscopy in infertility investigation. *Am. J. Obstet. Gynecol.*, **156**, 558–60.

Fedele, L., Brioschi, D., Dorta, M., Marchini, M., and Parazzini, F. (1988). Prediction and self-prediction of ovulation in clomiphene citrate-treated patients. *Eur. J. Obstet. Gynecol. Reprod. Biol.*, **28**, 297–303.

Fedorkow, D. M., Corenblum, B., Pattinson, H. A., and Taylor, P. J. (1988). Septuplet gestation following the use of human menopausal gonadotropin despite extensive monitoring. *Fertil. Steril.*, **49**, 364–6.

Feinstein, A. (1977). *Clinical biostatistics*, pp. 214–26. C. V. Mosby, St Louis.

Feuer, G. S. (1983). The psychological impact of infertility on the lives of men. *Dissertation Abstracts International*, 44, 706A–707A.

Filicori, M., Butler, J. P., and Crowley, jun., W. F. (1984). Neuroendocrine regulation of the corpus luteum in the human: evidence for pulsatile progesterone secretion. *J. Clin. Invest.*, 73, 1638–47.

Findlay, J. K. (1984). Implantation and early pregnancy. In In vitro *fertilization and embryo transfer* (ed. C. Trounson and C. Wood), pp. 57–72. Churchill Livingstone, Edinburgh.

Fisch, P., Casper, R. F., Brown, S. E., Wrixon, W., Collins, J. A., Reid, R., *et al.* (1989). Unexplained infertility: evaluation of treatment with clomiphene citrate and human chorionic gonadotropin. *Fertil. Steril.*, 51, 828–33.

Fleiss, J. L. (1981). *Statistical methods for rates and proportions*, 2nd edn, p. 56. Wiley, Toronto.

Fluhmann, C. F. (1961). *The cervix uteri and its diseases*. Saunders, Philadelphia.

Forsey, J. P. and Hull, M. G. R. (1989). Unexplained infertility. In *Recent advances in the management of infertility* (ed. C. Chen, S. L. Tan, and W. C. D. Cheng), pp. 27–66. McGraw-Hill, Singapore.

Fox, C. A. (1973). Recent studies in human coital physiology. *Clin. Endoc. Metab.*, 2, 527–43.

Francavilla, F., Catignani, P., Romano, R., Santucci, R., Francavilla, S., Poccia, G., *et al.* (1984). Immunological screening of a male population with infertile marriages. *Andrologia*, 16, 578–86.

Franco, J. G., Schimberni, M., and Stone, S. C. (1987). An immunobead assay for antibodies to spermatozoa in serum. *J. Reprod. Med.*, 32, 188–90.

Frank, R. (1950). A clinical study of 240 infertile couples. *Am. J. Obstet. Gynecol.*, 60, 645–54.

Frank, D. I. (1984). Counseling the infertile couple. *J. of Psych. Nurs. Men. Health Serv.*, 22(5), 17–23.

Franklin, R. R. and Dukes, C. D. (1964). Antispermatozoal antibody and unexplained infertility. *Am. J. Obstet. Gynecol.*, 89, 6–9.

Fraser, A. (1984). *The weaker vessel: women's lot in seventeenth-century England*, p. 63. Weidenfeld and Nicolson, London.

Freund, M. (1962). Interrelationships among the characteristics of human semen and factors affecting semen-specimen quality. *J. Reprod. Fertil.*, 4, 143–59.

Friberg, J. (1981a). Postcoital testing in relation to circulating sperm-agglutinating antibodies in women. *Am. J. Obstet. Gynecol.*, 139, 587–91.

Friberg, J. (1981*b*). Postcoital tests and sperm-agglutinating antibodies in men. *Am. J. Obstet. Gynecol.*, 141, 76–80.

Fritsch, H. (1894). Ein Fall von Volligen Schwund der Gebärmutterhohle nach Aufkratzung. *Centralblatt für Gynaecologie*, 52, 52–4.

Gabos, P. (1976). A comparison of hysterosalpingography and endoscopy in evaluation of tubal function in infertile women. *Fertil. Steril.*, 27, 238–42.

Gallinat, A. (1984). Hysteroscopy as a diagnostic and therapeutic procedure in sterility. In *Hysteroscopy principles and practice* (ed. A. M. Siegler and J. B. Lindemann), pp. 180–5. Lippincott, Philadelphia.

Garcia, J. E., Jones, G. S., and Wright, jun., G. L. (1981). Prediction of the time of ovulation. *Fertil. Steril.*, 36, 308–15.

Gellert-Mortimer, S. T., Clarke, G. N., Baker, H. W. G., Hyne, R. V., and Johnston, W. I. H. (1988). Evaluation of Nycondenz and Percoll density gradients for the selection of motile human spermatozoa. *Fertil. Steril.*, 49, 335–41.

Gemzell, C. (1977). Induction of ovulation with human gonadotropins. *J. Reprod. Med.*, 18, 155–8.

Gibor, Y., Garcia, jun., C. J., Cohen, M. R., and Scommegna, A. (1970). The cyclical changes in the physical properties of the cervical mucus and the results of the postcoital test. *Fertil. Steril.*, 21, 20–7.

Gilula, N. B., Fawcett, D. W., and Aoki, A. (1976). The sertoli cell occluding junctions and gap junctions in mature and developing mammalian testis. *Dev. Biol.*, 50, 142–68.

Gilula, N. B., Epstein, M. L., and Beers, W. H. (1978). Cell-to-cell communication and ovulation: a study of the cumulus–oocyte complex. *J. Cell. Biol.*, 78, 58–75.

Glass, R. H. and Ericsson, R. J. (1978). Intrauterine insemination of isolated motile sperm. *Fertil. Steril.*, 29, 535–8.

Glass, R. H. and Goldbus, M. S. (1978). Habitual abortion. *Fertil. Steril.*, 29, 257–65.

Glazener, C. M., Kelly, N. J., and Hull, M. G. (1987*a*). Prolactin measurement in the investigation of infertility in women with a normal menstrual cycle. *Br. J. Obstet. Gynaecol.*, 94, 535–8.

Glazener, C. M. A., Kelly, N. J., and Hull, M. G. R. (1987*b*). Borderline hyperprolactinemia in infertile women: evaluation of the prolactin response to thyrotropin-releasing hormone and double-blind placebo-controlled treatment with bromocriptine. *Gynecol. Endocrinol.*, 1, 373–8.

Glazener, C. M. A., Kelly, N. J., Weir, M. J. A., David, J. S. E., Cornes, J. S., and Hull, M. G. R. (1987*c*). The diagnosis of male infertility—prospective time-specific study of conception rates related to seminal analysis and post-coital sperm–mucus penetration and survival in otherwise unexplained infertility. *Hum. Reprod.*, 2, 665–71.

Glazener, C. M. A., Loveden, L. M., Richardson, S. J., Jeans, W. D., and Hull, M. G. R. (1987*d*). Tubo-cornual polyps: their relevance in subfertility. *Hum. Reprod.*, 2, 59–62.

Glazener, C. M. A., Kelly, N. J., and Hull, M. G. R. (1988). Luteal deficiency not a persistent cause of infertility. *Hum. Reprod.*, 3, 213–17.

Glazener, C. M. A., Coulson, C., Lambert, P. A., Watt, E. M., Hinton, R. A., Kelly, N. G., *et al.* (1990). Clomiphene treatment for women with unexplained infertility: placebo-controlled study of hormonal responses and conception rates. *Gynecol. Endocrinol.*, 4, 75–83.

Glazer, S. and Cooper, S. L. (1988). Moving on, or: when is enough enough? In *Without child* (ed. S. Glazer and S. L. Cooper), pp. 143–8. Lexington, Mass.

Gnarpe, H. and Friberg, J. (1972). *Mycoplasma* and human reproductive failure. I. The occurrence of different Myocoplasmas in couples with reproductive failure. *Am. J. Obstet. Gynecol.*, 114, 727–31.

Goldberg, J. M., Haering, P. L., Friedman, C. I., Dodds, W. G., and Kim, M. H. (1990). Antisperm antibodies in women undergoing intrauterine insemination. *Am. J. Obstet. Gynecol.*, 163, 65–8.

Goldenberg, R. L. and Magendantz, H. G. (1976). Laparoscopy and the infertility evaluation. *Obstet. Gynecol.*, 47, 410–14.

Goldstein, D., Zuckerman, H., Harpaz, S., Bakai, J., Geva, A., Gordon, S., *et al.* (1982). Correlation between estradiol and progesterone in cycles with luteal phase deficiency. *Fertil. Steril.*, 37, 348–54.

Gomel, V. and Taylor, P. J. (1986). The technique of endoscopy. In *Laparoscopy and hysteroscopy in gynaecologic practice* (ed. V. Gomel, P. J. Taylor, A. A. Yuzpe, and J. E. Rioux), p. 212. Yearbook Medical Publishers, Chicago.

Gomel, V., Taylor, P. J., Yuzpe, A. A., and Rioux, J. E. (1986). Indications, contraindications and complications. In *Laparoscopy and hysteroscopy in gynaecologic practice* (ed. V. Gomel, P. J. Taylor, A. A. Yuzpe, and J. E. Rioux), pp. 56–74. Yearbook Medical Publishers, Chicago.

Gonzales, J. and Jezequel, F. (1985). Influence of the quality of the cervical mucus on sperm penetration: comparison of the morphologic features of spermatozoa in 101 postcoital tests with those in the semen of the husband. *Fertil. Steril.*, 44, 796–9.

Gordts, S., Boeckx, W., Vasquez, G., and Brosens, I. (1983). Microsurgical resection of intramural tubal polyps. *Fertil. Steril.*, 40, 258–9.

Gotterer, G., Ginsberg, D., Schulman, T., Banks, J., and Williams-Ashman, H. G. (1955). Enzymatic coagulation of semen. *Nature*, 176, 1209–11.

Gould, S. F., Shannon, J. M., and Cunha, G. R. (1983). Nuclear estrogen binding sites in human endometriosis. *Fertil. Steril.*, 39, 520–4.

Gould, J. E., Overstreet, J. W., and Hanson, F. W. (1984). Assessment of human sperm function after recovery from the female reproductive tract. *Biol. Reprod.*, 31, 888–94.

Griffin, M. E. (1983). Resolving infertility: an emotional crisis. *AORN J*, 38, 597–601.

Griffith, C. S. and Grimes, D. A. (1990). The validity of the postcoital test. *Am. J. Obstet. Gynecol.*, 162, 616–20.

Grinstead, J., Jacobsen, J. D., Grinsted, L., Schantz, A., Stenfoss, H. H., and Nielsen, S. P. (1989). Prediction of ovulation. *Fertil. Steril.*, 52, 388–93,

Gump, D. W., Gibson, M., and Ashikaga, T. (1984). Lack of association between genital mycoplasmas and infertility. *New Engl. J. Med.*, 310, 937–41.

Gwatkin, R. B. L., Collins, J. A., Jarrell, J. F., Kohut, J., and Milner, R. A. (1990). The value of semen analysis and sperm function assays in predicting pregnancy among infertile couples. *Fertil. Steril.*, 53, 693–9.

Haas, G. (1985). Clarifying antibody-mediated infertility. *Am. J. Reprod. Immunol. Microbiol.*, 7, 148.

Haas, G. G. and Cunningham, M. E. (1984). Identification of antibody-laden sperm by cytofluorometry. *Fertil. Steril.*, 42, 606–13.

Haas, G. G., Cines, D. B., and Schreiber, A. D. (1980). Immunologic infertility: identification of patients with antisperm antibody. *New Engl. J. Med.*, 303, 722–7.

Haas, G. G., Schreiber, A. D., and Blasco, L. (1983). The incidence of sperm-associated immunoglobulin and C3, the third component of complement, in infertile men. *Fertil. Steril.*, 39, 542–7.

Haas, G. G., D'Cruz, O. J., and DeBault, L. E. (1991). Comparison of the indirect immunobead, radiolabeled, and immunofluorescence assays for immunoglobulin G serum antibodies to human sperm. *Fertil. Steril.*, 55, 377–88.

Hackeloer, B. J. (1978). Ultrasonic demonstration of follicular development. *Lancet*, i, 941.

Hafez, E. S. E. (1973). Gamete transport. In *Human reproduction, conception and contraception* (ed. E. S. E. Hafez and T. N. Evans), pp. 85–118. Harper and Row, New York.

Hafez, E. S. E. (1980). The cervix in sperm transport. In *Human repro-*

duction, conception and contraception, 2nd edn (ed. E. S. E. Hafez), pp. 221–52. Harper and Row, New York.

Halbert, S. A. (1983). Function and structure of the fallopian tube. In *Microsurgery in female infertility* (ed. V. Gomel), pp. 7–27. Little, Brown, Boston.

Halbert, S. A. and Patton, D. L. (1981). Ovum pick-up following fimbriectomy and infundibular salpingostomy in rabbits. *J. Reprod. Med.*, **26**, 299–307.

Halme, J., Hammond, M. G., Hulka, J. F., Raj, S. G., and Talbert, L. M. (1984*a*). Retrograde menstruation in healthy women and in patients with endometriosis. *Obstet. Gynecol.*, **64**, 151–4.

Halme, J., Becker, S., and Wing, R. (1984*b*). Accentuated cyclic activation of peritoneal macrophages in patients with endometriosis. *Am. J. Obstet. Gynecol.*, **148**, 85–90.

Hamilton, A. (1792). *A treatise on the management of female complaints*, p. 146. Peter Hill, Edinburgh.

Hamilton, C. J. C. M., Evers, J. L. H., and de Haan, J. (1986). Ultrasound increases the prognostic value of the postcoital test. *Gynecol. Obstet. Invest.*, **21**, 80–8.

Hamou, J. (1981). Microhysteroscopy. A new procedure and its original applications in gynecology. *J. Reprod. Med.*, **26**, 375–82.

Hamou, J. and Taylor, P. J. (1982). Panoramic, contact, and micro-colpohysteroscopy in gynaecologic practice. *Curr. Prob. Obstet. Gynecol.*, **2**, 1–18.

Hanafiah, M. J., Epstein, J. A., and Sobrero, A. J. (1972). Sperm-agglutinating antibodies in 236 infertile couples. *Fertil. Steril.*, **23**, 493–7.

Hancock, R. J. T. and Faruki, S. (1984). Detection of antibody-coated sperm by 'panning' procedures. *J. Immunol. Meth.*, **66**, 149–59.

Handelsman, D. J., Conway, A. J., Radonic, I., and Turtle, J. R. (1983). Prevalence, testicular function and seminal parameters in men with sperm antibodies. *Clin. Reprod. Fertil.*, **2**, 39–45.

Haney, A. F., Muscato, J. J., and Weinberg, J. B. (1981). Peritoneal fluid cell populations in infertility patients. *Fertil. Steril.*, **35**, 696–8.

Haney, A. F., Misukonis, M. A., and Weinberg, J. B. (1983). Macrophages and infertility: oviductal macrophages as potential mediators of infertility. *Fertil. Steril.*, **39**, 310–15.

Hansson, V., Djoseland, O., Reusch, E., Attramadal, A., and Torgersen, O. (1973). An androgen-binding protein in the testis cytosol fraction of adult rats. Comparison with the androgen-binding protein in the epididymis. *Steroids*, **21**, 457–74.

Hargreave, T. (1982). Incidence of serum agglutinating and immobilizing sperm antibodies in infertile couples. *Int. J. Fertil.*, **27**, 90–4.

Hargreave, T. B. and Elton, R. A. (1986). Fecundability rates from an infertile male population. *Br. J. Urol.*, **58**, 194–7.

Hargreave, T. B., Aitken, R. J., and Elton, R. A. (1988). Prognostic significance of the zona-free hamster egg test. *Br. J. Urol.*, **62**, 603–8.

Hargrove, J. T. and Abraham, G. E. (1980). Abnormal luteal function in endometriosis. *Fertil. Steril.*, **34**, 302.

Harrison, R. F. (1980). Pregnancy successes in the infertile couple. *Int. J. Fertil.*, **25**, 81–7.

Harrison, R. F. (1981). The diagnostic and therapeutic potential of the postcoital test. *Fertil. Steril.*, **36**, 71–5.

Harrison, R. F., O'Moore, R. R., and McSweeney, J. (1979). Idiopathic infertility: a trial of bromocriptine versus placebo. *Irish Med. J.*, **72**, 479–82 (Abstract).

Hartz, S. C., Medical Research International, Society for Assisted Reproductive Technology, and The American Fertility Society (1991). *In vitro* fertilization–embryo transfer (IVF–ET) in the United States: 1989 results from the IVF–ET registry. *Fertil. Steril.*, **55**, 14–23.

Hearn, J. P., Gidley-Baird, A. A., Hodges, J. K., Summers, P. M., and Webley, G. E. (1988). Embryonic signals during the peri-implantation period in primates. *J. Reprod. Fert. Suppl.*, **36**, 49–58.

Hecht, B. R., Khan-Dawood, F. S., and Dawood, M. Y. (1989). The luteinizing hormone surge: timing and characteristics in the plasma and urine after clomiphene citrate treatment. *Fertil. Steril.*, **52**, 401–5.

Heller, C. G. and Clairmont, Y. (1963). Spermatogenesis in man: an estimate of its duration. *Science*, **140**, 184–6.

Hellstrom, W. J. G., Schachter, J., Sweet, R. L., and McClure, R. D. (1987). Is there a role for *Chlamydia trachomatis* and genital *Mycoplasma* in male infertility? *Fertil. Steril.*, **48**, 337–9.

Heniger, J. (1973). Leeuwenhoek, Antoni Van. In *Dictionary of scientific biography, Vol. VIII* (ed. J. H. Lane and P. J. Macquer), pp. 126–30. Scribner, New York.

Herman, A., Ron-El, R., Golan, A., Raziel, A., Soffer, Y., and Caspi, E. (1990). Pregnancy rate and ovarian hyperstimulation after luteal human chorionic gonadotropin in *in vitro* fertilization stimulated with gonadotropin-releasing hormone analog and menotropins. *Fertil. Steril.*, **53**, 92–6.

Hirschowitz, J. S., Soler, N. G., and Wortsman, J. (1978). The galactorrhoea–endometriosis syndrome. *Lancet*, **i**, 896–8.

Hjort, T., Johnson, P. M., and Mori, T. (1985). An overview of the WHO international multi-centre study on antibodies to reproductive tract antigens in clinically defined sera. *J. Reprod. Immun.*, **8**, 359–62.

Ho, P.-C., Poon, I. M. L., Chan, S. Y. W., and Wang, C. (1989). Intrauterine insemination is not useful in oligoasthenospermia. *Fertil. Steril.*, **51**, 682–4.

Honea-Fleming, P. A. and Honea, K. L. (1984). Psychological locus of control in infertile women. *Fertil. Steril.*, **41**, 96S–97S (Abstract).

Horne, H. W. and Thibault, J. P. (1962). Sperm migration through the human female reproductive tract. *Fertil. Steril.*, **13**, 135–9.

Horvath, P. M., Beck, M., Bohrer, M. K., Shelden, R. M., and Kemmann, E. (1989). A prospective study on the lack of development of antisperm antibodies in women undergoing intrauterine insemination. *Am. J. Obstet. Gynecol.*, **160**, 631–7.

Howe, S. E., Grider, S. L., Lynch, D. M., and Fink, L. M. (1991). Antisperm antibody binding to human acrosin: a study of patients with unexplained infertility. *Fertil. Steril.*, **55**, 1176–82.

Huang, K.-E. (1986). The primary treatment of luteal phase inadequacy: progesterone versus clomiphene citrate. *Am. J. Obstet. Gynecol.*, **155**, 824–8.

Hughes, E. G., Collins, J. P., and Garner, P. R. (1987). Homologous artificial insemination for oligoasthenospermia: a randomized controlled study comparing intracervical and intrauterine techniques. *Fertil. Steril.*, **48**, 278–81.

Hull, M. G. R., Savage, P. E., Bromham, D. R., Ismail, A. A. A., and Morris, A. F. (1982a). The value of a single serum progesterone measurement in the midluteal phase as a criterion of a potentially fertile cycle ('ovulation') derived from treated and untreated conception cycles. *Fertil. Steril.*, **37**, 355–60.

Hull, M. G. R., Savage, P. E., and Bromham, D. R. (1982b). Prognostic value of the postcoital test: prospective study based on time-specific conception rates. *Br. J. Obstet. Gynecol.*, **89**, 299–305.

Hull, M. G. R., Glazener, C. M. A., Kelly, N. J., Conway, D. I., Foster, P. A., Hinton, R. A., *et al.* (1985). Population study of causes, treatment, and outcome of infertility. *Br. Med. J.*, **291**, 1693–7.

Hull, M. E., Moghissi, K. S., Magyar, D. F., and Hayes, M. F. (1987). Comparison of different treatment modalities of endometriosis in infertile women. *Fertil. Steril.*, **47**, 40–4.

Hunt, R. B. and Siegler, M. A. (1990). *Hysterosalpingography techniques and interpretation*, p. 186. Yearbook Medical Publishers, Chicago.

Hunter, R. H. F. (1987). Human fertilization *in vivo* with special reference to progression, storage and release of competent spermatozoa. *Hum. Reprod.*, **2**, 329–32.

Husted, S. and Hjort, T. (1975). Microtechnique for simultaneous determination of immobilizing and cytotoxic sperm antibodies: methodological and clinical studies. *Clin. Exp. Immunol.*, **22**, 256–64.

Huszar, G., Corrales, M., and Vigue, L. (1988). Correlation between sperm creatine phosphokinase activity and sperm concentrations in normospermic and oligospermic men. *Gamete Res.*, **19**, 67–75.

Hutchins, C. J. (1977). Laparoscopy and hysterosalpingography in the assessment of tubal patency. *Obstet. Gynecol.*, **49**, 325–7.

Hutchinson-Williams, K. A., Decherney, A. H., Lavy, G., Diamond, M. P., Naftolin, F., and Lunenfeld, B. (1990). Luteal rescue in *in vitro* fertilization–embryo transfer. *Fertil. Steril.*, **53**, 495–501.

Idris, W. and Jewelewicz, R. (1976). A comparative study of hysterosalpingography and laparoscopy in the investigation of infertility. *Int. J. Gynaecol. Obstet.*, **14**, 428–30.

Iffland, C. A., Shaw, R. W., and Beynon, J. L. (1989). Is danazol a useful treatment in unexplained primary infertility? *Eur. J. Obstet. Gynecol. Reprod. Biol.*, **32**, 115–21.

Iffland, C. A., Reid, W., Amso, N., Bernard, A. G., Buckland, G., and Shaw, R. W. (1991). A within-patient comparison between superovulation with intra-uterine artificial insemination using husband's washed spermatozoa and gamete intrafallopian transfer in unexplained infertility. *Eur. J. Obstet. Gynecol. Reprod. Biol.*, **39**, 181–6.

Ingerslev, H. J. and Ingerslev, M. (1980). Clinical findings in infertile women with circulating antibodies against spermatozoa. *Fertil. Steril.*, **33**, 514–20.

Insler, V., Melmed, H., Eichenbrenner, I., Serr, D. M., and Lunenfeld, B. (1972). The cervical score: a simple semiquantitative method for monitoring of the menstrual cycle. *Int. J. Gynaecol. Obstet.*, **10**, 223–8.

Insler, V., Potashnik, G., and Glassner, M. (1981). Some epidemiological aspects of fertility evaluation. In *Advances in diagnosis and treatment of infertility* (ed. V. Insler, G. Bettendorf, and K.-H. Geissler), pp. 165–77. Elsevier–North Holland, New York.

Irvine, D. S. and Aitken, R. J. (1985). The value of adenosine triphosphate (ATP) measurements in assessing the fertilizing ability of human spermatozoa. *Fertil. Steril.*, **44**, 806–13 (Abstract).

Ismajovich, B., Wexler, S., Golan, A., Langer, L., and David, M. P. (1986). The accuracy of hysterosalpingography versus laparoscopy in evaluation of infertile women. *Int. J. Gynaecol. Obstet.*, **24**, 9–12.

Isojima, S., Tsuchiya, K., Koyama, K., Tanaka, C., Naka, O., and Adachi, H. (1972). Further studies on sperm-immobilizing antibody found in sera of unexplained cases of sterility in women. *Am. J. Obstet. Gynecol.*, **112**, 199–207.

Jager, S., Kremer, J., and Kiuken, J. (1977). Immunoglobulin classes of sperm antibodies in cervical mucus. In *Immunologic influence on human fertility* (ed. B. Boettcher), pp. 289–93. Sydney Academic Press, Sydney.

Jager, S., Kremer, J., and Van Slochteren-Draaisma, T. (1978). A simple method of screening for antisperm antibodies in the human male. Detection of spermatozoal surface IgG with the direct mixed antiglobulin reaction carried out on untreated fresh human semen. *Int. J. Fertil.*, **23**, 12–21.

Jager, S., Kremer, J., and De Wilde-Janssen, I. (1984). Are sperm-immobilizing antibodies in cervical mucus an explanation for a poor postcoital test? *Am. J. Reprod. Immunol.*, **5**, 56–60.

James, W. (1979). The causes of the decline in fecundability with age. *Soc. Biol.*, **26**, 330–3.

Jansen, R. P. S. (1978). Fallopian tube isthmic mucus and ovum transport. *Science*, **201**, 349–51.

Jansen, R. P. S. (1980). Cyclic changes in the human fallopian tube isthmus and their functional importance. *Am. J. Obstet. Gynecol.*, **136**, 292–308.

Jansen, R. and Russell, P. (1986). Non-pigmented endometriosis: clinical, laparascopic, and pathologic definition. *Am. J. Obstet. Gynecol.*, **155**, 1154–9.

Jansen, R. P. S., Anderson, J. C., Radonic, I., Smit, J., and Sutherland, P. D. (1988). Pregnancies after ultrasound-guided fallopian insemination with cryostored donor semen. *Fertil. Steril.*, **49**, 920–2.

Jennings, M. G., McGowan, M. P., and Baker, H. W. (1985). Immunoglobulins on human sperm: validation of a screening test for sperm autoimmunity. *Clin. Reprod. Fertil.*, **3**, 335–42.

Jequier, A. M. (1986). *Current reviews in obstetrics and gynecology No. 11: Infertility in the Male*, pp. 1–154. Churchill Livingstone, New York.

Jette, N. T. and Glass, R. H. (1972). Prognostic value of the postcoital test. *Fertil. Steril.*, **23**, 29–32.

Johansson, C.-J. (1957). Clinical studies on sterile couples with special reference to the diagnosis, etiology and prognosis of infertility. *Acta Obstet. Gynecol. Scand.*, **36** (Suppl. 5), 1–168.

Jones, G. E. S. (1949). Some newer aspects of the management of infertility. *JAMA*, **141**, 1123–9.

Joyce, C. R. B., Last, J. M., and Weatherall, M. (1968). Personal factors as a cause of differences in prescribing by general practitioners. *Br. J. Prev. Soc. Med.*, **22**, 170–7.

Kane, J. L., Woodland, R. M., Forsey, T., Darougar, S., and Elder,

M. G. (1984). Evidence of chlamydial infection in infertile women with and without fallopian tube obstruction. *Fertil. Steril.*, 42, 843–8.

Kaplan, C. R., Olive, D. L., Sabella, V., Asch, R. H., Balmaceda, J. P., Riehl, R. M., *et al.* (1989). Gamete intrafallopian transfer vs superovulation with intrauterine insemination for the treatment of infertility. *J. In Vitro Fert. Embryo Transf.*, 6, 298–304.

Karacagil, M., Imamoglu, A., Pasaoglu, H., Gulmez, I., and Tatlisen, A. (1989). The effect of spermine, spermidine and kallikrein on the triple adenosine triphosphatase enzyme activity of spermatozoa in males with oligoasthenozoospermia. *Br. J. Urol.*, 63, 84–6.

Katz, D. F. and Overstreet, J. W. (1980). Mammalian sperm movement in the secretions of the male and female genital tract. In *Testicular development, structure and function* (ed. A. Steinberger and E. Steinberger), pp. 481–9. Raven Press, New York.

Keirse, M. J. N. C. and Vandervellen, R. (1973). A comparison of hysterosalpingography and laparoscopy in the investigation of infertility. *Obstet. Gynecol.*, 41, 685–8.

Keller, D. W., Strickler, R. C., and Warren, J. C. (1984). Fundamental considerations. In *Clinical infertility*, (ed. D. W. Keller, R. C. Strickler, and J. C. Warren), pp. 2–3. Appleton–Century Crofts, Norwalk, Connecticut.

Kerin, J. F. P., Peek, J., Warnes, G. M., Kirby, C., Jeffrey, R., Matthews, C. D., *et al.* (1984). Improved conception rate after intrauterine insemination of washed spermatozoa from men with poor-quality semen. *Lancet*, i, 533–5.

Khatamee, M. A. and Decker, W. H. (1978). Recovery of genital mycoplasmas from infertile couples using New York City medium. *Infertility*, 1, 155–8.

Kirby, C. A., Flaherty, S. P., Godfrey, B. M., Warnes, G. M., and Matthews, C. D. (1991). A prospective trial of intrauterine insemination of motile spermatozoa versus timed intercourse. *Fertil. Steril.*, 56, 102–7.

Kistner, R. W. (1975). Induction of ovulation with clomiphene citrate. In *Progress in infertility*, 2nd edn (ed. S. J. Behrman and R. W. Kistner), pp. 509–36. Little, Brown, Boston.

Kjaergaard, N., Mortensen, B. B., Hostrup, P., and Lauritsen, J. G. (1990). Prognostic value of semen analyses in infertility evaluation (male fertility/life-table analysis). *Andrologia*, 22, 62–8.

Kliger, B. E. (1984). Evaluation, therapy, and outcome in 493 infertile couples. *Fertil. Steril.*, 41, 40–6.

Knee, G. R., Feinman, M. A., Strauss III, J. F., Blasco, L., and Goodman, D. B. P. (1985). Detection of the ovulatory luteinizing hormone (LH) surge with a semiquantitative urinary LH assay. *Fertil. Steril.*, **44**, 707–9.

Knobil, E. (1980). The neuroendocrine control of the menstrual cycle. *Recent Prog. Horm. Res.*, **36**, 53–88.

Kobayashi, S., Bessho, T., Shigeta, M., Koyama, K., and Isojima, S. (1990). Correlation between quantitative antibody titers of sperm-immobilizing antibodies and pregnancy rates by treatments. *Fertil. Steril.*, **54**, 1107–13.

Koninckx, P. R., Ide, P., Vandenbroucke, W., and Brosens, I. A. (1978). New aspects of the pathophysiology of endometriosis and associated infertility. *J. Reprod. Med.*, **24**, 257–60.

Kossoy, L. R., Hill, G. A., Herbert, C. M., Brodie, B. L., Dalglish, C. S., Dupont, W. D., *et al.* (1988). Therapeutic donor insemination: the impact of insemination timing with the aid of a urinary luteinizing hormone immunoassay. *Fertil. Steril.*, **49**, 1026–9.

Kovacs, G. T., Newman, G. B., and Henson, G. L. (1978). The post-coital test: what is normal? *Br. Med. J.*, **1**, 818.

Kremer, J. (1965). A simple sperm penetration test. *Int. J. Fertil.*, **10**, 209–15.

Kremer, J. (1968). Sperm penetration in cervical mucus. In *Fertility investigation, Thesis 24*. Drukkerij Van Denderen N.V., Groningen, Holland.

Kurzrok, R. and Miller, E. G. (1928). Biochemical studies of human semen and its relation to mucus of the cervix uteri. *Am. J. Obstet. Gynecol.*, **15**, 56–72.

Kusuda, M., Nakamura, G., Matsukuma, K., and Kurano, A. (1983). Corpus luteum insufficiency as a cause of nidatory failure. *Acta Obstet. Gynecol. Scand.*, **62**, 199–205.

Labastida, R., Dexeus, S., and Arias, A. (1988). Infertility and hysteroscopy. In *Hysteroscopy principles and practice* (ed. A. M. Siegler and H. J. Lindemann), pp. 175–9. Lippincott, Philadelphia.

Ladipo, O. A. (1976). Tests of tubal patency: comparison of laparoscopy and hysterosalpingography. *Br. Med. J.*, **2**, 1297–8.

Lalos, A., Lalos, O., Jacobsson, L., and von Schoultz, B. (1985). A psychosocial characterization of infertile couples before surgical treatment of the female. *J. Psychosom. Obstet. Gynecol.*, **4**, 83.

Landgren, B.-M., Unden, A.-L., and Diczfalusy, E. (1980). Hormonal profile of the cycle in 68 normally menstruating women. *Acta Endocrinol.*, **94**, 89–98.

Leader, A., Wiseman, D., and Taylor, P. J. (1985). The prediction of ovulation: a comparison of the basal body temperature graph, cervical mucus score, and real-time pelvic ultrasonography. *Fertil. Steril.*, **43**, 385–8.

Lee, R. L. and Lipschultz, L. I. (1985). Evaluation and treatment of male infertility. In *Infertility: a practice guide for the physician*, 2nd edn (ed. M. G. Hammond and L. M. Talbert), pp. 42–63. Medical Economics Books, New Jersey.

Leeton, J. and Kerin, J. (1984). Embryo transfer. In *Clinical* in vitro *fertilization* (ed. C. Wood and A. Trounson), pp. 116–36. Springer-Verlag, Berlin.

Leeton, J., Mahadevan, M., Trounson, A., and Wood, C. (1984). Unexplained infertility and the possibilities of management with *in vitro* fertilization and embryo transfer. *Aust. NZ J. Obstet. Gynaec.*, **24**, 131–4.

Leeton, J., Rogers, P., Caro, C., Healy, D., and Yates, C. (1987). A controlled study between the use of gamete intrafallopian transfer (GIFT) and *in vitro* fertilization and embryo transfer in the management of idiopathic and male infertility. *Fertil. Steril.*, **48**, 605–7.

Lemay, A., Maheux, R., Huot, C., Blanchet, J., and Faure, N. (1988). Efficacy of intranasal or subcutaneous luetinizing hormone-releasing hormone agonist inhibition of ovarian function in the treatment of endometriosis. *Am. J. Obstet. Gynecol.*, **158**, 233–6.

Lenton, E. A., Weston, G. A., and Cooke, I. D. (1977). Long-term follow-up of the apparently normal couple with a complaint of infertility. *Fertil. Steril.*, **28**, 913–19.

Lenton, E. A., Neal, L. M., and Sulaiman, R. (1982). Plasma concentrations of human chorionic gonadotropin from the time of implantation until the second week of pregnancy. *Fertil. Steril.*, **37**, 773–8.

Lenton, E. A., Landgren, B.-M., and Sexton, L. (1984). Normal variation in the length of the luteal phase of the menstrual cycle: identification of the short luteal phase. *Br. J. Obstet. Gynaecol.*, **91**, 685–9.

Levin, R. M., Shofer, J., Wein, A. J., and Greenberg, S. H. (1981). ATP concentration of human spermatozoa: lack of correlation with sperm motility. *Andrologia*, **13**, 468–72.

Levinson, C. J. (1989). Endometriosis therapy: rationale for expectant or minimal therapy in minimal/mild cases (AFSI). *Proceedings—2nd World Congress of Gynecologic Endoscopy, Clermont-Ferrand, France, June 5–8* (Abstract).

Lewinthal, D., Taylor, P. J., Pattinson, H. A., and Corenblum, B. (1988). Induction of ovulation with luprolide acetate and human menopausal gonadotropin. *Fertil. Steril.*, **49**, 585–8.

Li, T.-C., Rogers, A., Lenton, E., Dockery, P., and Cooke, I. (1987). A comparison between two methods of chronological dating of human endometrial biopsies during the luteal phase, and their correlation with histologic dating. *Fertil. Steril.*, **48**, 928–32.

Li, T.-C., Dockery, P., Rogers, A. W., and Cooke, I. D. (1989). How precise is histologic dating of endometrium using the standard dating criteria? *Fertil. Steril.*, **51**, 759–63.

Li, T.-C., Dockery, P., and Cooke, I. D. (1991). Endometrial development in the luteal phase of women with various types of infertility: comparison with women of normal fertility. *Hum. Reprod.*, **6**, 325–30.

Lindemann, H.-J. (1979). CO_2-hysteroscopy today. *Endoscopy*, **2**, 94–100.

Link, P. W. and Darling, C. A. (1986). Couples undergoing treatment for infertility: dimensions of life satisfaction. *J. Sex Marital Therapy*, **12**, 46–59.

Lippes, J., Enders, R. G., Pragay, D. A., and Bartholomew, W. R. (1972). The collection and analysis of human fallopian tubal fluid. *Contraception*, **5**, 85–103.

Liston, W. A., Bradford, W. P., Downie, J., and Kerr, M. G. (1972). Laparoscopy in a general gynecologic unit. *Am. J. Obstet. Gynecol.*, **113**, 672–7.

Lorton, S. P., Kummerfield, H. L., and Foote, R. H. (1981). Polyacrylamide as a substitute for cervical mucus in sperm migration tests. *Fertil. Steril.*, **35**, 222–5.

Lubke, F. and Hindenburg, H.-J. (1984). Hysteroscopy as an examination method in sterility. In *Hysteroscopy principles and practice*, (ed. A. M. Siegler and H. J. Lindemann), pp. 173–4. Lippincott, Philadelphia.

Lukse, M. P. (1985). The effect of group counseling on the frequency of grief reported by infertile couples. *Journal of Obstetric and Gynecologic Nursing*, **14** (Suppl. 6), 67s–70s.

Lundquist, F. (1949). Aspects of the biochemistry of human semen. *Acta Physiol. Scand.* **19** (Suppl 66), 5–105.

Lunenfeld, B. and Lunenfeld, E. (1990). Ovulation induction: HMG. In *Infertility, a comprehensive text* (ed. M. M. Siebel), pp. 311–22. Appleton and Lange, Norwalk, Connecticut.

Lynch, D. M., Leali, B. A., and Howe, S. E. (1986). A comparison of sperm agglutination and immobilization assays with a quantitative ELISA for anti-sperm antibody in serum. *Fertil. Steril.*, **46**, 285–92.

Lyons, E. A., Ballard, G., Taylor, P. J., Levi, C. S., Zheng, S. H., and Kredentser, J. V. (1991). Characterization of subendometrial myometrial contractions throughout the menstrual cycle in normal fertile women. *Fertil. Steril.*, **55**, 771–4.

Maathuis, J. B. and Aitken, R. J. (1978). Cyclic variation in concentrations of protein and hexose in human uterine flushings collected by an improved technique. *J. Reprod. Fertil.*, **52**, 289–95.

Maathuis, J. B., Horbach, J. G. M., and van Hall, E. V. (1972). A comparison of the results of hysterosalpingography and laparoscopy in the diagnosis of fallopian tube dysfunction. *Fertil. Steril.*, **23**, 428–31.

Maathuis, J. B., Van Look, P. F. A., and Michie, E. A. (1978). Changes in volume, total protein and ovarian steroid concentrations of peritoneal fluid throughout the human menstrual cycle. *J. Endocrinol.*, **76**, 123–33.

McArdle, C. R. and Berezin, A. F. (1980). Ultrasound demonstration of uterus subseptus. *J. Clin. Ultrasound*, **8**, 139–41.

McBain, J. C. and Pepperell, R. J. (1982). Use of bromocriptine in unexplained infertility. *Clin. Reprod. Fertil.*, **1**, 145–50.

McIntosh, J. E. A., Matthews, C. D., Crocker, J. M., Broom, T. J., and Cox, L. W. (1980). Predicting the luteinizing hormone surge: relationship between the duration of the follicular and luteal phases and the length of the human menstrual cycle. *Fertil. Steril.*, **34**, 125–30.

MacLeod, J. (1964). Human seminal cytology as a sensitive indicator of the germinal epithelium. *Int. J. Fertil.*, **9**, 281–95.

MacLeod, J. and Gold, R. Z. (1953). The male factor in fertility and infertility. VI. Semen quality and certain other factors in relation to ease of conception. *Fertil. Steril.*, **4**, 10–33.

Macnamee, M. C., Howles, C. M., Edwards, R. G., Taylor, P. J., and Elder, K. T. (1989). Short-term luteinizing hormone-releasing hormone agonist treatment: prospective trial of a novel ovarian stimulation regimen for *in vitro* fertilization. *Fertil. Steril.*, **52**, 264.

McNatty, K. P., Sawers, R. S., and McNeilly, A. S. (1974). A possible role for prolactin in control of steroid secretion by human Graafian follicle. *Nature*, **250**, 653–5.

Macomber, D. and Sanders, M. B. (1929). The spermatozoa count: its value in the diagnosis, prognosis, and treatment of sterility. *New Engl. J. Med.*, **200**, 981–4.

Magyar, D. M., Boyers, S. P., Marshall, J. R., and Abraham, G. E. (1979). Regular menstrual cycles and premenstrual molimina as indicators of ovulation. *Obstet. Gynecol.*, **53**, 411–14.

Mahadevan, M. M. and Trounson, A. O. (1984). The influence of seminal characteristics on the success rate of human *in vitro* fertilization. *Fertil. Steril.*, **42**, 400–5.

Mahlstedt, P. P. (1985). The psychological component of infertility. *Fertil. Steril.*, **43**, 335–46.

Mahmood, T. A. and Templeton, A. (1991). Prevalence and genesis of endometriosis. *Hum. Reprod.*, **6**, 544–9.

Mai, F. M., Munday, R. N., and Rump, E. E. (1972). Psychiatric interview comparisons between infertile couples. *Psychosom. Med.*, **34**, 431–40.

Maia, H. S. and Coutinho, E. M. (1972). Peristalsis and antiperistalsis of the human fallopian tube during the menstrual cycle. *Biol. Reprod.*, **2**, 305–14.

Mancini, R. E., Andrada, J. A., Saraceni, D., Bachmann, A. E., Lavieri, J. C., and Nemirovsky, M. (1965). Immunological and testicular response in man sensitized with human testicular homogenate. *J. Clin. Endocrinol. Metab.*, **25**, 859–75.

Mandelbaum, S. L., Diamond, M. P., and DeCherney, A. (1987). Relationship of antisperm antibodies to oocyte fertilization in *in vitro* fertilization–embryo transfer. *Fertil. Steril.*, **47**, 644–51.

Manotaya, T. and Potter, E. L. (1963). Oocytes in prophase of meiosis from squash preparations of human fetal ovaries. *Fertil. Steril.*, **14**, 378–92.

Mantel, N. (1966). Evaluation of survival data and two new rank order statistics arising in its consideration. *Cancer Chemother. Rep.*, **50**, 163–70.

Mao, C. and Grimes, D. A. (1988). The sperm penetration assay: can it discriminate between fertile and infertile men? *Am. J. Obstet. Gynecol.*, **159**, 279–86.

Maranna, R., Lucisano, A., Leone, F., Sanna, A., Dell'Acqua, S., and Mancuso, S. (1990). High prevalence of silent chlamydia colonization of the tubal mucosa in infertile women. *Fertil. Steril.*, **53**, 354–9.

Mardh, P.-A., Westrom, L., von Mecklenburg, C., and Hammar, E. (1976). Studies on ciliated epithelia of the human genital tract. I. Swelling of the cilia of the fallopian tube epithelium in organ cultures infected with *Mycoplasma hominis*. *Br. J. Vener. Dis.*, **52**, 52–7.

Marik, J. and Hulka, J. (1978). Luteinized unruptured follicle syndrome: a subtle cause of infertility. *Fertil. Steril.*, **29**, 270–4.

Marshak, R. H., Poole, C. S., and Goldberger, M. A. (1950). Hysterography and hysterosalpingography. *Surg. Gynecol. Obstet.*, **91**, 182–92.

Marshall, J. (1963). Thermal changes in the normal menstrual cycle. *Br. Med. J.*, **1**, 102–4.

Marshall, J. R. (1970). Ovulation induction. *Obstet. Gynecol.*, **35**, 963–70.

Martin, D. C., Hubert, G. D., Vander Zwaag, R., and El-Zeky, F. A. (1989). Laparoscopic appearances of peritoneal endometriosis. *Fertil. Steril.*, **51**, 63–7.

Martinez, F., Trounson, A., and Besanko, M. (1986). Detection of the LH surge for AID, AIH and embryo transfer using a twice daily urinary dipstick assay. *Clin. Reprod. Fertil.*, 4, 45–53.

Martinez, A. R., Bernardus, R. E., Voorhorst, F. J., Vermeiden, J. P. W., and Schoemaker, J. (1991). Pregnancy rates after timed intercourse or intrauterine insemination after human menopausal gonadotropin stimulation of normal ovulatory cycles: a controlled study. *Fertil. Steril.*, 55, 258–65.

Maruyama, jun., D. K., Hale, R. W., and Rogers, B. J. (1985). Effects of white blood cells on the *in vitro* penetration of zona-free hamster eggs by human spermatozoa. *J. Androl.*, 6, 127–35.

Masui, Y. and Clarke, H. J. (1979). Oocyte maturation. *Int. Rev. Cytol.*, 57, 185–282.

Mathur, S., Baker, E. R., Williamson, H. O., Derrick, F. C., Teague, K. J., and Fudenberg, H. H. (1981). Clinical significance of sperm antibodies in infertility. *Fertil. Steril.*, 36, 486–95.

Mathur, S., Peress, M. R., Williamson, H. O., Youmans, C. D., Maney, S. A., Garvin, A. J., *et al.* (1982). Autoimmunity to endometrium and ovary in endometriosis. *Clin. Exp. Immunol.*, 50, 259–66.

Mathur, S., Williamson, H. O., Baker, M. E., Rust, P. F., Holtz, G. L., and Fudenberg, H. H. (1984). Sperm motility on postcoital testing correlates with male autoimmunity to sperm. *Fertil. Steril.*, 41, 81–7.

Mattler, P. E. (1973). The cervix and its secretions in relation to fertility and ruminence. In *The biology of the cervix* (ed. R. J. Blandau and K. S. Moghissi), pp. 339–50. University of Chicago Press.

Meinertz, H. and Hjort, T. (1986). Detection of autoimmunity to sperm: mixed antiglobulin reaction (MAR) test or sperm agglutination? A study on 537 men from infertile couples. *Fertil. Steril.*, 46, 86–91.

Menge, A. C. and Fleming, C. H. (1978). Detection of sperm antigens on mouse ova and early embryos. *Dev. Biol.*, 63, 111–17.

Menge, A. C., Medley, N. E., Mangione, C. M., and Dietrich, J. W. (1982). The incidence and influence of antisperm antibodies in infertile human couples on sperm–cervical mucus interactions and subsequent fertility. *Fertil. Steril.*, 38, 439–46.

Menken, J., Trussell, J., and Larsen, U. (1986). Age and infertility. *Science*, 26, 1389–94.

Menning, B. E. (1977). *Infertility: a guide for the childless couple.* Prentice-Hall, Englewood Cliffs, NJ.

Menning, B. E. (1982). The psychosocial impact of infertility. *Nurs. Clin. North Am.*, 17, 155–63.

Menon, N., Peegel, H., and Katta, V. (1985). Estradiol potentiation of gonadotropin-releasing hormone responsiveness in the anterior pituitary is mediated by an increase in gonadotrophin-releasing hormone receptors. *Am. J. Obstet. Gynecol.*, **151**, 534–40.

Meyer, R. (1919). Ober den stand der grage der adenomyositis und adneomyome in allgemeinen und insbesondere über adenomyositis serosoepithelialis und adenomyometritis sacromatosa. *Abl. f. Gynäk.*, **43**, 745–6.

Miller, E. G. and Kurzrok, R. (1932). Biochemical studies of human semen. III. Factors affecting migration of sperm through the cervix. *Am. J. Obstet. Gynecol.*, **24**, 19–26.

Moghissi, K. S. (1976a). Accuracy of basal body temperature for ovulation detection. *Fertil. Steril.*, **27**, 1415–21.

Moghissi, K. S. (1976b). Postcoital test: physiologic basis, technique, and interpretation. *Fertil. Steril.*, **27**, 117–28 (Abstract).

Moghissi, K. S. (1984). The function of the cervix in human reproduction. *Curr. Probl. Obstet. Gynecol. Fertil.*, **7**(3), 23–41.

Moghissi, K. S. and Sim, G. S. (1975). Correlation between hysterosalpingography and pelvic endoscopy for the evaluation of tubal factor. *Fertil. Steril.*, **26**, 1178–81.

Moghissi, K. S., Dabich, D., Levine, J., and Neuhaus, O. W. (1964). Mechanism of sperm migration. *Fertil. Steril.*, **15**, 15–23.

Moghissi, K. S., Sacco, A. G., and Borin, K. (1980). Immunologic infertility. I. Cervical mucus antibodies and postcoital test. *Am. J. Obstet. Gynecol.*, **136**, 941–50.

Mohr, L. R. (1984). Assessment of human embryos. In *In vitro fertilization and embryo transfer* (ed. A. Trounson and C. Wood), pp. 159–71. Churchill Livingstone, Edinburgh.

Mohr, L. R. and Trounson, A. (1984). *In vitro* fertilization and embryo growth. In *Clinical in vitro fertilization* (ed. C. Wood and A. Trounson), pp. 99–115. Springer-Verlag, Berlin.

Mohr, L. R., Trounson, A., Leeton, J. F., and Wood, C. (1983). Evaluation of normal and abnormal human embryo development during procedures *in vitro*. In *Fertilization of the human egg in vitro: biological basis and clinical application* (ed. H. M. Beier and H. R. Lindner), pp. 211–21. Springer-Verlag, Berlin.

Monif, G. R. G. (1990). Infections. In *Infertility, a comprehensive text* (ed. M. M. Siebel), pp. 235–40. Appleton and Lange, Norwalk, Connecticut.

Moore, D. E., Foy, H. M., Daling, J. R., Grayston, J. T., Spadoni, L. R., Wang, S. P., *et al.* (1982). Increased frequency of serum antibodies to *Chlamydia trachomatis* in infertility due to distal tubal disease. *Lancet*, **ii**, 574–7.

Morales, P., Katz, D. F., Overstreet, J. W., Samuels, S. J., and Chang, R. J. (1988). The relationship between the motility and morphology of spermatozoa in human semen. *J. Androl.*, **9**, 241–7.

Morris, N. M., Underwood, L. E., and Easterling, W. (1976). Temporal relationship between basal body temperature nadir and luteinizing hormone surge in normal women. *Fertil. Steril.*, **27**, 780–3.

Mortimer, D. (1983). Sperm transport in human female reproductive tract. In *Oxford reviews of reproductive biology*, Vol. 5 (ed. C. A. Finn), pp. 31–61. Clarendon Press, Oxford.

Mortimer, D. (1985*a*). The male factor in infertility. Part I. Semen analysis. *Curr. Probl. Obstet. Gynecol. Fertil.*, **8**(7), 1–87.

Mortimer, D. (1985*b*). The male factor in infertility. Part II. Sperm function testing. *Curr. Probl. Obstet. Gynecol. Fertil.*, **8**(8), 1–75.

Mortimer, D. and Templeton, A. A. (1982). Sperm transport in the human female reproductive tract in relation to semen analysis characteristics and time of ovulation. *J. Reprod. Fert.*, **64**, 401–8.

Mortimer, D., Shu, M. A., and Tan, R. (1986). Standardization and quality control of sperm concentration and sperm motility counts in semen analysis. *Hum. Reprod.*, **1**, 299–303.

Mortimer, D., Curtis, E. F., Camenzind, A. R., and Tanaka, S. (1989). The spontaneous acrosome reaction of human spermatozoa incubated *in vitro*. *Hum. Reprod.*, **4**, 57–62.

Morton, H., Rolfe, B. E., McNeill, L., Clarke, P., Clarke, F. M., and Clunie, G. J. A. (1980). Early pregnancy factor: tissues involved in its production in the mouse. *J. Reprod. Immunol.*, **3**, 73–82.

Moszkowski, E., Woodruff, J. D., and Jones, G. E. S. (1962). The inadequate luteal phase. *Am. J. Obstet. Gynecol.*, **83**, 363–72.

Moudgal, N. R., Moyle, W. R., and Greep, R. O. (1971). Specific binding of luteinizing hormone of Leydig tumor cells. *J. Biol. Chem.*, **246**, 4983–6.

Murdoch, A. P., Harris, M., Mahroo, M., Williams, M., and Dunlop, W. (1991). Is GIFT (gamete intrafallopian transfer) the best treatment for unexplained infertility? *Br. J. Obstet. Gynecol.*, **98**, 643–7.

Murphy, A. A., Guzick, D. S., and Rock, J. A. (1989). Microscopic peritoneal endometriosis. *Fertil. Steril.*, **51**, 1072–3.

Muscato, J. J., Haney, A. F., and Weinberg, J. B. (1982). Sperm phagocytosis by human peritoneal macrophages: a possible cause of infertility in endometriosis. *Am. J. Obstet. Gynecol.*, **144**, 503–10 (Abstract).

Muse, K. N. and Wilson, E. A. (1982). How does mild endometriosis cause infertility? *Fertil. Steril.*, **38**, 145–52.

Nachtigall, R. D., Faure, N., and Glass, R. H. (1979). Artificial insemination of husband's sperm. *Fertil. Steril.*, **32**, 141–7.

Newton, J., Craig, S., and Joyce, D. (1974). The changing pattern of a comprehensive infertility clinic. *J. Biosoc. Sci.*, **6**, 477–82.

Nilsson, S., Edvinsson, A., and Nilsson, B. (1979). Improvement of semen and pregnancy rate after ligation and division of the internal spermatic vein: fact or fiction? *Br. J. Urol.*, **51**, 591–6.

Nisolle, M., Paindaveine, B., Bourdon, A., Berliere, M., Casanas-Roux, F., and Donnez, J. (1990). Histologic study of peritoneal endometriosis in infertile women. *Fertil. Steril.*, **53**, 984–8.

Nordenskjold, F. and Ahlgren, M. (1983). Laparoscopy in female infertility: diagnosis and prognosis for subsequent pregnancy. *Acta Obstet. Gynecol. Scand.*, **62**, 609–15.

Novy, M. J. (1980). Reversal of Kroener fimbriectomy sterilization. *Am. J. Obstet. Gynecol.*, **137**, 198–206.

Noyes, R. W., Hertig, A. T., and Rock, J. A. (1950). Dating the endometrial biopsy. *Fertil. Steril.*, **1**, 3–25.

Odem, R. R., Durso, N. M., Long, C. A., Pineda, J. A., Strickler, R. C., and Gast, M. J. (1991). Therapeutic donor insemination: a prospective randomized study of scheduling methods. *Fertil. Steril.*, **55**, 976–82.

O'Herlihy, C., De Crespigny, L. J. Ch., and Robinson, H. P. (1980). Monitoring ovarian follicular development with real-time ultrasound. *Br. J. Obstet. Gynaecol.*, **87**, 613–18.

Olive, D. L., Weinberg, J. B., and Haney, A. F. (1985). Peritoneal macrophages and infertility: the association between cell number and pelvic pathology. *Fertil. Steril.*, **44**, 772–7.

Orrell, K. G. S., Wrixon, W., and Irwin, A. C. (1980). The clinical prediction of ovulation. *Nova Scotia Med. Bull.*, **59**, 119–21.

Osborn, J. C. and Moor, R. M. (1982). Cell interactions and ACTIN synthesis in mammalian oocytes. *J. Exp. Zool.*, **220**, 125–9.

Overstreet, J. (1986). Evaluation of sperm–cervical mucus interaction. *Fertil. Steril.*, **45**, 324–6.

Pandya, I. J., Mortimer, D., and Sawers, R. S. (1986). A standardized approach for evaluating the penetration of human spermatozoa into cervical mucus *in vitro*. *Fertil. Steril.*, **45**, 357–65.

Papanicolaou, G. N. (1946). A general survey of the vaginal smear and its use in research and diagnosis. *Am. J. Obstet. Gynecol.*, **51**, 316–28.

Pattinson, H. A., Mortimer, D., and Taylor, P. J. (1990). Treatment of sperm agglutination with proteolytic enzymes II. Sperm function after enzymatic disagglutination. *Hum. Reprod.*, **5**, 174–8.

Pauerstein, C. J., Turner, T., and Eddy, C. A. (1977). A technique for evaluating functional patency of the oviduct. *Fertil. Steril.*, **28**, 777–80.

Peng, H.-Q., Collins, J. A., Wilson, E. H., and Wrixon, W. (1987). Receiver-operating characteristics curves for semen analysis variables: methods for evaluating diagnostic tests of male gamete function. *Gamete Res.*, **17**, 229–36.

Perloff, W. H. and Steinberger, E. (1963). *In vitro* penetration of cervical mucus by spermatozoa. *Fertil. Steril.*, **14**, 231–6.

Petrie, A. (1982). The crossover design. In *The randomized clinical trial and therapeutic decisions* (ed. N. Tygstrup, J. M. Lachin, and E. Juhl), pp. 199–204. Marcel Dekker, New York.

Philipsen, T. and Hansen, B. B. (1981). Comparative study of hysterosalpingography and laparoscopy in infertile patients. *Acta Obstet. Gynecol. Scand.*, **60**, 149–51.

Phillips, J., Keith, D., Hulka, J., Hulka, B., and Keith, L. (1976). Gynecological laparoscopy in 1975. *J. Reprod. Med.*, **16**, 105–17.

Pittaway, D. E., Maxson, W., Daniell, J., Herbert, C., and Wentz, A. (1983). Luteal phase defects in infertility patients with endometriosis. *Fertil. Steril.*, **39**, 712–13.

Polansky, F. F. and Lamb, E. J. (1989). Analysis of three laboratory tests used in the evaluation of male fertility: Bayes' rule applied to the postcoital test, the *in vitro* mucus migration test, and the zona-free hamster egg test. *Fertil. Steril.*, **51**, 215–28.

Portuondo, J. A., Echanojauregui, A. D., Irala, J. P., and Calonge, J. (1980). Triple evaluation of tubal patency. *Int. J. Fertil.*, **25**, 307–10.

Portuondo, J. A., Barral, A., Melchor, J. C., Tanago, J. G., and Neyro, J. L. (1984). Chromosomal complements in primary gonadal failure. *Obstet. Gynecol.*, **64**, 757–61.

Prader, A. (1966). Testicular size: assessment and clinical importance. *Triangle*, 7, 240–3.

Pretorius, E. and Franken, D. (1989). The predictive value of the postcoital test for auto- and isoimmunity to spermatozoa. *Andrologia*, **21**, 584–8 (Abstract).

Quagliarello, J. and Arny, M. (1986). Inaccuracy of basal body temperature charts in predicting urinary luteinizing hormone surges. *Fertil. Steril.*, **45**, 334–7.

Queenan, J. T., O'Brien, G. D., Bains, L. M., Simpson, J., Collins, W. P., and Campbell, S. (1980). Ultrasound scanning of ovaries to detect ovulation in women. *Fertil. Steril.*, **34**, 99–105.

Radwanska, E., Hammond, J., and Smith, P. (1981). Single midluteal progesterone assay in the management of ovulatory infertility. *J. Reprod. Med.*, **26**, 85–9.

Ragni, G., Lombroso, G. C., Bestetti, O., De Laurextis, L., and Agosti, S. (1984). Hysteroscopy versus hysterosalpingography in infertile patients. *Int. J. Fertil.*, **29**, 141–2.

Ramsewak, S. S., Barratt, C. L. R., Li, T.-C., Gooch, H., and Cooke, I. D. (1990). Peritoneal sperm recovery can be consistently demonstrated in women with unexplained infertility. *Fertil. Steril.*, **53**, 1106–8.

Ramzy, I. (1983). *Essentials of gynecologic and obstetric pathology*, pp. 166–9. Appleton-Century Crafts, Norwalk, Connecticut.

Raymont, A., Arronet, G. H., and Arrata, W. S. M. (1969). Review of 500 cases of infertility. *Int. J. Fertil.*, **14**, 141–53.

Riad-Fahmy, D., Read, G. F., Walker, R. F., Walker, S. M., and Griffiths, K. (1987). Determination of ovarian steroid hormone levels in saliva. *J. Reprod. Med.*, **32**, 254–72.

Rice, J. P., London, S. S. N., and Olive, D. L. (1986). Re-evaluation of hysterosalpingography in infertility investigation. *Obstet. Gynecol.*, **67**, 718–21.

Richards, J. S. (1980). Maturation of ovarian follicles: action and interactions of pituitary and ovarian hormones on follicular cell differentiation. *Physiol. Rev.*, **60**, 51–89.

Ridley, J. H. (1968). The histogenesis of endometriosis. A review of facts and fancies. *Obstet. Gynecol. Surv.*, **23**, 1–35.

Ritchie, A. W. S., Hargreave, T. B., James, K., and Chisholm, G. D. (1984). Intra-epithelial lymphocytes in the normal epididymis: a mechanism for tolerance to sperm auto-antigens? *Br. J. Urol.*, **56**, 79–83.

Robarts, P. and Braude, P. (1987). Variations in ambient temperature can lead to incorrect prediction of the luteinizing hormone surge using urinary dipsticks (OvuSTICK). *Br. J. Obstet. Gynaecol.*, **94**, 486–7.

Rock, J. and Bartlett, M. K. (1937). Biopsy studies of human endometrium: criteria of dating and information about amenorrhea, menorrhagia and time of ovulation. *JAMA*, **108**, 2022–8.

Roddick, jun., J. W., Conkey, G., and Jacobs, E. J. (1960). The hormonal response of endometrium in endometriotic implants and its relationship to symptomatology. *Am. J. Obstet. Gynecol.*, **79**, 1173–7.

Rodgers-Neame, N. T., Garrison, P. N., Younger, J. B., and Blackwell, R. E. (1986). Determination of antisperm antibodies in infertile couples by Millititer filtration. *Fertil. Steril.*, **45**, 299–301.

Rodriguez-Rigau, L. J., Smith, K. D., and Steinberger, E. (1978). Relationship of varicocele sperm to output and fertility of male partners in infertile couples. *J. Urol.*, **120**, 691–4.

Rose, N. R., Hjort, T., Rumke, P., Harper, M. J. K., and Vyazov, O. (1976). Techniques for detection of iso and auto antibodies to human spermatozoa. *Clin. Exp. Immunol.*, **23**, 175–99.

Rosenberg, S. M., Luciano, A. A., and Riddick, D. H. (1980). The luteal phase defect: the relative frequency of, and encouraging response to, treatment with vaginal progesterone. *Fertil. Steril.*, 34, 17–20.

Rosenfeld, D. L. and Garcia, C. R. (1976). A comparison of endometrial histology with simultaneous plasma progesterone determinations in infertile women. *Fertil. Steril.*, 27, 1256–66.

Rosenfeld, D. L. and Mitchell, E. (1979). Treating the emotional aspects of infertility: counseling services in an infertility clinic. *Am. J. Obstet. Gynecol.*, 135, 177–80.

Rosenfeld, D. L., Chudow, S., and Bronson, R. A. (1980). Diagnosis of luteal phase inadequacy. *Obstet. Gynecol.*, 56, 193–6.

Rosenfeld, D. L., Seidman, S. M., Bronson, R. A., and Scholl, G. M. (1983). Unsuspected chronic pelvic inflammatory disease in the infertile female. *Fertil. Steril.*, 39, 44–8.

Rousseau, S., Lord, J., Lepage, Y., and Van Campenhout, J. (1983). The expectancy of pregnancy for 'normal' infertile couples. *Fertil. Steril.*, 40, 768–72.

Rowland, G. F., Forsey, T., Moss, T. R., Steptoe, P. C., Hewitt, J., and Darougar, S. (1985). Failure of *in vitro* fertilization and embryo replacement following infection with *Chlamydia trachomatis. J IVF ET*, 2, 151–5.

Rubin, I. C. (1921). Subphrenic pneumoperitoneum produced by intra-uterine insufflation of oxygen as a test of patency of the fallopian tubes in sterility and in allied gynecological conditions. *Am. J. Roentgenol.*, 8, 120–8.

Rubinstein, B. B. (1937). The relation of cyclic changes in human vaginal smears to body temperatures and basal metabolic rates. *Am. J. Physiol.*, 119, 635–41.

Ruijs, G. F., Kauer, F. M., Jager, S., Schroder, F. P., Schirm, J., and Kremer, J. (1990). Is serology of any use when searching for correlations between *Chlamydia trachomatis* infection and male infertility? *Fertil. Steril.*, 53, 131–6.

Ruijs, G. J., Kauer, F. M., Jager, S., Schroder, F. P., Schirm, J., and Kremer, J. (1991). Further details on sequelae at the cervical and tubal level of *Chlamydia trachomatis* infection in infertile women. *Fertil. Steril.*, 56, 20–6.

Rumke, P. H. (1974). The origin of immunoglobulins in semen. *Clin. Exp. Immunol.*, 17, 287–97.

Rumke, P. H. and Hellinga, G. (1959). Autoantibodies against spermatozoa in sterile men. *Am. J. Clin. Path.*, 32, 357–63.

Rumke, P. H., Renckens, C. N. M., Bezemer, P. D., and Van Amstel,

N. (1984). Prognosis of fertility in women with unexplained infertility and sperm agglutinins in the serum. *Fertil. Steril.*, **42**, 561–7.

Salat-Baroux, J., Maillard, G., Verges, P., Hamou, J. E., and Chouraqui, A. (1984). Complications from microhysteroscopy. In *Hysteroscopy, principles and practice* (ed. A. M. Siegler and H. J. Lindemann), pp. 112–18. Lippincott, Philadelphia.

Samburg, I., Martin-du-pan, R., and Bourrit, B. (1985). The value of the postcoital test according to etiology and outcome of infertility. *Acta Eur. Fertil.*, **16**, 147–9.

Sampson, J. A. (1925). Heterotopic or misplaced endometrial tissue. *Am. J. Obstet. Gynecol.*, **10**, 649–64.

Sampson, J. A. (1927). Peritoneal endometriosis due to the menstrual dissemination of endometrial tissue into the peritoneal cavity. *Am. J. Obstet. Gynecol.*, **14**, 422–69.

Sandow, J., Fraser, H. M., and Geisthovel, F. (1986). Pharmacology and experimental basis of therapy with LHRH agonists in women. *Prog. Clin. Biol. Res.*, **225**, 1–27.

SanFillippo, J. S., Yussman, M. A., and Smith, O. (1978). Hysterosalpingography in the evaluation of infertility: a six-year review. *Fertil. Steril.*, **30**, 636–43.

Santomauro, A. G., Sciarra, J. J., and Varma, A. O. (1972). A clinical investigation of the role of the semen analysis and postcoital test in the evaluation of male infertility. *Fertil. Steril.*, **23**, 245–51.

Sarrel, P. M. and DeCherney, A. H. (1985). Psychotherapeutic intervention for treatment of couples with secondary infertility. *Fertil. Steril.*, **43**, 897–900.

Sarris, S., Swyer, G. I. M., McGarrigle, H. H. G., Lawrence, D. M., Little, V., and Lachelin, G. C. L. (1978). Prolactin and luteal insufficiency. *Clin. Endocrinol.*, **9**, 543–7.

Sathananthan, A. H. (1984). Ultrastructure morphology of fertilization and early cleavage in the human. In *In vitro fertilization and embryo transfer* (ed. A. Trounson and C. Wood), pp. 131–58. Churchill Livingstone, Edinburgh.

Sathananthan, A. H. and Trounson, A. O. (1982). Ultrastructure of cortical granule release and zona interaction in monospermic and polyspermic human ova fertilization *in vitro*. *Gamete Res.*, **6**, 225–34.

Sawatzky, M. (1981). Tasks of infertile couples. *Journal of Obstetric and Gynecologic Nursing.*, **10**, 132–3.

Schats, R., Aitken, R., Templeton, A. A., and Djahanbakhch, O. (1984). The role of cervical mucus–semen interaction in infertility of unknown aetiology. *Br. J. Obstet. Gynaecol.*, **91**, 371–6.

Schenken, R. S. and Malinak, L. R. (1982). Conservative surgery versus expectant management for the infertile patient with mild endometriosis. *Fertil. Steril.*, **37**, 183–6.

Schmidt, C. L. (1985). Endometriosis: a reappraisal of pathogenesis and treatment. *Fertil. Steril.*, **44**, 157–73.

Schoenfeld, C., Amelar, R. D., and Dubin, L. (1976). Clinical experience with sperm antibody testing. *Fertil. Steril.*, **27**, 1199–203.

Schumacher, G. F. B. (1980). Humoral immune factors in the female reproductive tract and their changes during the cycle. In *Immunologic aspects of infertility and fertility regulation* (ed. D. Dhindsa and G. F. B. Schumacher), pp. 93–142. Elsevier, New York.

Schwabe, M. G., Shapiro, S. S., and Haning, jun., R. V. (1983). Hysterosalpingography with oil contrast medium enhances fertility in patients with infertility of unknown etiology. *Fertil. Steril.*, **40**, 604–6.

Schwartz, D. and Mayaux, M. J. (1982). Female fecundability as a function of age: results from artificial insemination in 2193 nulliparous women with azoospermic husbands. *New Engl. J. Med.*, **306**, 404–6.

Schweppe, K.-W. (1988). Etiology, pathogenesis and natural history of endometriosis. In *Recent advances in the management of endometriosis* (ed. J. A. Rock and K.-W. Schweppe), pp. 13–30. Parthenon Publishing Group, Carnforth, Lancs.

Schweppe, K.-W. and Wynn, R. M. (1981). Ultrastructural changes in endometriotic implants during the menstrual cycle. *Obstet. Gynecol.*, **58**, 465–73.

Sciarra, J. J. and Valle, R. F. (1977). Hysteroscopy: a clinical experience with 320 patients. *Am. J. Obstet. Gynecol.*, **127**, 340–8.

Scott, R. T., Snyder, R. R., Strickland, D. M., Tyburski, C. C., Bagnall, J. A., Reed, K. R., *et al.* (1988). The effect of interobserver variation in dating endometrial histology on the diagnosis of luteal phase defects. *Fertil. Steril.*, **50**, 888–92.

Seastrunk, J. W., Kemery, T. D., Adelsberg, B., McCaskill, C., and Bellina, J. H. (1984). Psychological evaluation of couples in an inpatient reproductive biology unit. *Fertil. Steril.*, **41**, 96S Suppl. (Abstract).

Seibel, M. and Taymor, M. (1982). Emotional aspects of infertility. *Fertil. Steril.*, **37**, 137–46.

Seibel, M. M. (1990). Work up of the infertile couple. In *Infertility: a comprehensive text* (ed. M. M. Seibel), pp. 1–22. Appleton and Lange, Norwalk, Connecticut.

Serafini, P., Stone, B., Kerin, J., Batzofin, J., Quinn, P., and Marrs, R. P. (1988). An alternate approach to controlled ovarian hyperstimulation in 'poor responders': pretreatment with a gonadotropin-releasing hormone analog. *Fertil. Steril.*, **49**, 90–5.

Serhal, P. F., Katz, M., Little, V., and Woronowski, H. (1988). Unexplained infertility—the value of pergonal superovulation combined with intrauterine insemination. *Fertil. Steril.*, 49, 602–6.

Servy, E. J. and Tzingounis, V. A. (1978). Tubal patency: hysterosalpingography compared with laparoscopy. *Southern Med. J.*, 71, 1511–12.

Setchell, B. P. and Jacks, F. (1974). Inhibin-like activity in rat testicular fluid. *J. Endocrinol.*, 62, 675–6.

Settlage, D. S. F., Motoshima, M., and Tredway, D. R. (1973). Sperm transport from the external cervical os to the fallopian tubes in women: a time and quantitation study. *Fertil. Steril.*, 24, 655–61.

Shabanowitz, R. B. and O'Rand, M. G. (1988). Molecular changes in the human zona pellucida associated with fertilization and human sperm–zona interactions. *Ann. NY Acad. Sci.*, 541, 621–32.

Shaffer, W. (1986). Role of uterine adhesions in the cause of multiple pregnancy losses. *Clin. Obstet. Gynecol.*, 29, 912–24.

Shalev, J., Goldenberg, M., Kukiae, E., Lewinthal, D., Tepper, R., Maschiach, S., *et al.* (1989). Comparison of five clomiphene citrate dosage regimes: follicular recruitment and distribution in human ovary. *Fertil. Steril.*, 52, 560–3.

Shangold, M., Berkeley, A., and Gray, J. (1983). Both midluteal serum progesterone levels and late luteal endometrial histology should be assessed in all infertile women. *Fertil. Steril.*, 40, 627–30.

Shaw, G. Bernard (1923). *The Doctor's Dilemma: A Tragedy*, pp. 6–7. Constable, London.

Shepard, M. K. and Senturia, Y. D. (1977). Comparison of serum progesterone and endometrial biopsy for confirmation of ovulation and evaluation of luteal function. *Fertil. Steril.*, 28, 541–8.

Sherins, R. J., Brightwell, D., and Sternthal, P. M. (1977). Longitudinal analysis of semen of fertile and infertile men. In *The testis in normal and infertile men* (ed. P. Troen and H. R. Nankin), pp. 473–88. Raven Press, New York.

Sherman, B. M., West, J. H., and Korenman, S. G. (1976). The menopausal transition: analysis of LH, FSH, estradiol and progesterone concentrations during menstrual cycles in older women. *J. Clin. Endocrinol. Metab.*, 42, 629–36.

Short, R. V. (1979). When a conception fails to become a pregnancy. In *Maternal recognition of pregnancy* (ed. J. M. Whelan), pp. 377–94. Excerpta Medica, Amsterdam.

Shoupe, D., Mishell, jun., D. R., Lacarra, M., Lobo, R. A., Horenstein, J., d'Ablaing, G., *et al.* (1989). Correlation of endometrial maturation with four methods of estimating day of ovulation. *Obstet. Gynecol.*, 73, 88–92.

Shy, K. K., Stenchever, M. A., and Muller, C. H. (1988). Sperm penetration assay and subsequent pregnancy: a prospective study of 74 infertile men. *Obstet. Gynecol.*, **71**, 685–90.

Silander, T. (1963). Hysteroscopy through a transparent rubber balloon in patients with carcinoma of the uterine endometrium. *Acta Obstet. Gynecol. Scand.*, **42**, 284–310.

Simpson, J. L., Elias, S., Malinak, L. R., and Buttram, jun., V. C. (1980). Heritable aspects of endometriosis: I. Genetic studies. *Am. J. Obstet. Gynecol.*, **137**, 327–31.

Sims, J. M. (1869). On the microscope as an aid in the diagnosis and treatment of sterility. *New York Med. Bull.*, **8**, 393–413.

Singer, S. L., Lambert, H., Cross, N. L., and Overstreet, J. W. (1985). Alteration of the human sperm surface during *in vitro* capacitation as assessed by lectin-induced agglutination. *Gamete Res.*, **12**, 291–9.

Small, D. R. J., Collins, J. A., Wilson, E. H., and Wrixon, W. (1987). Interpretation of semen analysis among infertile couples. *Can. Med. Assoc. J.*, **136**, 829–33.

Smith, K. D., Rodriguez-Rigau, L. J., and Steinberger, E. (1977). Relation between indices of semen analysis and pregnancy rate in infertile couples. *Fertil. Steril.*, **28**, 1314–19.

Snowden, E. U., Jarrett II, J. C., and Dawood, M. Y. (1984). Comparison of diagnostic accuracy of laparoscopy, hysteroscopy, and hysterosalpingography in evaluation of female infertility. *Fertil. Steril.*, **41**, 709–13.

Soffer, Y., Marcus, Z., Bukovsky, I., and Caspi, E. (1976). Immunological factors and postcoital test in unexplained infertility. *Int. J. Fertil.*, **21**, 89–95.

Soffer, Y., Ron-El, R., Golan, A., Herman, A., Caspi, E., and Samra, Z. (1990). Male genital mycoplasmas and *Chlamydia trachomatis* culture: its relationship with accessory gland function, sperm quality, and autoimmunity. *Fertil. Steril.*, **53**, 331–6.

Solter, D. and Schachner, M. (1976). Brain and sperm cell surface antigen (NS-4) on preimplantation mouse embryos. *Dev. Biol.*, **52**, 98–104.

Sorensen, S. S. (1980). Infertility factors: their relative importance and share in an unselected material of infertility patients. *Acta Obstet. Gynecol. Scand.*, **59**, 513–20.

Southam, A. L. (1960). What to do with the 'normal' infertile couple? *Fertil. Steril.*, **11**, 543–9.

Southam, A. L. and Buxton, L. (1956). Seventy postcoital tests made during the conception cycle. *Fertil. Steril.*, **7**, 133–40.

Southam, A. L. and Buxton, C. L. (1957). Factors influencing reproductive potential. *Fertil. Steril.*, **8**, 25–35.

Spencer, L. (1987). Male infertility: psychological correlates. *Post Grad. Med.*, **81**, 223–8.

Speroff, L., Glass, R. H., and Kase, N. G. (1989*a*). Neuroendocrinology. In *Clinical gynecologic endocrinology and infertility*, 4th edn, pp. 15–89. Williams and Wilkins, Baltimore.

Speroff, L., Glass, R. H., and Kase, N. G. (1989*b*). The ovary from conception to senescence. In *Clinical gynecologic endocrinology and infertility*, 4th edn, pp. 121–63. Williams and Wilkins, Baltimore.

Stalheim, O. H. V., Proctor, S. J., and Gallagher, J. E. (1976). Growth and effects of ureaplasmas (T-myocoplasmas) in bovine oviductal organ cultures. *Infect. Immun.*, **13**, 915–25.

Stanwell-Smith, R. and Hendry, W. (1984). The prognosis of male subfertility: a survey of 1025 men referred to a fertility clinic. *Br. J. Urol.*, **56**, 422–8.

Steele, R. W., Dmowski, W. P., and Marmer, D. J. (1984). Immunologic aspects of human endometriosis. *Am. J. Reprod. Immunol.*, **6**, 33–6.

Steinberger, E. (1971). Hormonal control of mammalian spermatogenesis. *Physiol. Rev.*, **51**, 1–22.

Steinberger, A., Heindel, J. J., and Lindsay, J. N. (1975). Isolation and culture of FSH responsive Sertoli cells. *Endocr. Res. Commun.*, **2**, 261–72.

Steptoe, P. C. (1967). *Laparoscopy in gynaecology*. Livingstone, Edinburgh.

Steptoe, P. C. and Edwards, R. G. (1978). Birth after the reimplantation of a human embryo. *Lancet*, ii, 366.

Stillman, R. J. (1982). *In utero* exposure to diethylstilbestrol: adverse effects on the reproductive tract and reproductive performance in male and female offspring. *Am. J. Obstet. Gynecol.*, **142**, 905–21.

Stumpf, P. G. and March, C. M. (1980). Febrile morbidity following hysterosalpingography: identification of risk factors and recommendations for prophylaxis. *Fertil. Steril.*, **33**, 487–92.

Styler, M. and Shapiro, S. S. (1985). Mollicutes (*Mycoplasma*) in infertility. *Fertil. Steril.*, **44**, 1–12.

Sugimoto, O. (1978). Diagnostic and therapeutic hysteroscopy for traumatic intrauterine adhesions. *Am. J. Obstet. Gynecol.*, **131**, 539–47.

Sutherland, P. D., Matson, P. L., Moore, H. D. M., Goswamy, R., Parsons, J. H., Vaid, P., *et al.* (1985). Clinical evaluation of the heterologous oocyte penetration (HOP) test. *Br. J. Urol.*, **57**, 233–6.

Swerdloff, R. S., Overstreet, J. W., Sokol, R. Z., and Rajfer, J. (1985). Infertility in the male. *Ann. Int. Med.*, **103**, 906–19.

Swolin, K. and Rosencrantz, M. (1972). Laparoscopy vs. hysterosalpingography in sterility investigations. A comparative study. *Fertil. Steril.*, **23**, 270–3.

Takahashi, K., Nagata, H., Abu Musa, A., Shibukawa, A., Yamasaki, H., and Kitao, M. (1990). Clinical usefulness of CA-125 levels in the menstrual discharge of patients with endometriosis. *Fertil. Steril.*, **54**, 360–2.

Tauber, P. F. and Zaneveld, L. J. D. (1976). Coagulation and liquifaction of human semen. In *Human semen and fertility regulation in men*, 2nd edn (ed. E. S. E. Hafez), pp. 153–66. C.V. Mosby, St Louis.

Taylor, P. J. (1985). The case against HSG as a first-line procedure. *Contemp. Obstet. Gynecol.*, **25**, 49–71.

Taylor, P. J. (1990). When is enough enough? *Fertil. Steril.*, **54**, 772–3.

Taylor, P. J. and Cumming, D. C. (1979). Laparoscopy in the infertile female. *Curr. Probl. Obstet. Gynecol.*, **2**, 3–59.

Taylor, P. J. and Gomel, V. (1986). Endoscopy in the infertile patient. In *Laparoscopy and hysteroscopy in gynaecologic practice* (ed. V. Gomel, P. J. Taylor, A. A. Yuzpe, and J. E. Rioux), pp. 75–94. Yearbook Medical Publishers, Chicago.

Taylor, P. and Graham, G. (1982). Is diagnostic curettage harmful in women with unexplained infertility? *Br. J. Obstet. Gynecol.*, **89**, 296–8.

Taylor, P. J. and McEwan, K. L. (1986). Patient- versus physician-rated prognosis of conception in tubal surgery candidates. *Infertility*, **9**, 106–17.

Taylor, P., Cumming, D., and Hill, P. (1981). Significance of intrauterine adhesions detected hysteroscopically in eumenorrheic infertile women and role of antecedent curettage in their formation. *Am. J. Obstet. Gynecol.*, **139**, 239–42.

Taylor, P. J., Lewinthal, D., Leader, A., and Pattinson, H. A. (1987). A comparison of Dextran 70 with carbon dioxide as the distention medium for hysteroscopy in patients with infertility or requesting reversal of a prior tubal sterilization. *Fertil. Steril.*, **47**, 861–3.

Taylor-Robinson, D. and McCormack, W. M. (1979). Mycoplasmas in human genitourinary infections. In *The mycoplasmas, Vol. II* (ed. J. C. Tully and R. F. Whitcomb), pp. 307–66. Academic Press, New York.

Telang, M., Reyniak, J. V., and Shulman, S. (1978). Antibodies to spermatozoa. VIII. Correlation of sperm antibody activity with post-coital tests in infertile couples. *Int. J. Fertil.*, **23**, 200–6.

Telimaa, S. (1988). Danazol and medroxyprogesterone acetate inefficacious in the treatment of infertility in endometriosis. *Fertil. Steril.*, **50**, 872–5.

Templeton, A. A. and Kerr, M. G. (1977). An assessment of laparoscopy as the primary investigation in the subfertile female. *Br. J. Obstet. Gynaecol.*, **84**, 760–2.

Templeton, A. A. and Mortimer, D. (1980). Laparoscopic sperm recovery in infertile women. *Br. J. Obstet. Gynaecol.*, **87**, 1128–31.

Templeton, A. A. and Mortimer, D. (1982). The development of a clinical test of sperm migration to the site of fertilization. *Fertil. Steril.*, **37**, 410–15.

Templeton, A. A. and Penney, G. C. (1982). The incidence, characteristics, and prognosis of patients whose infertility is unexplained. *Fertil. Steril.*, **37**, 175–82.

teVelde, E. R., van Kooy, R. J., and Waterreus, J. J. H. (1989). Intrauterine insemination of washed husband's spermatozoa: a controlled study. *Fertil. Steril.*, **51**, 182–5.

Thibault, C. (1972). Physiology and physiopathology of the fallopian tube. *Int. J. Fertil.*, **17**, 1–13.

Thomas, E. J. and Cooke, I. D. (1987). Successful treatment of asymptomatic endometriosis: does it benefit infertile women? *Br. Med. J.*, **294**, 1117–19.

Thomas, A. K. and Forrest, M. S. (1980). Infertility: a review of 291 infertile couples over eight years. *Fertil. Steril.*, **34**, 106–11.

Tietze, C. (1956). Statistical contributions to the study of human fertility. *Fertil. Steril.*, **7**, 88–95.

Torode, H. W., McPetrie, R. A., Wheeler, P. A., Metcalf, S. C., Saunders, D. M. and Ackerman, V. P. (1987). The role of chlamydial antibodies in an *in vitro* fertilization programme. *Fertil. Steril.*, **48**, 987–90.

Tredway, D. R., Buchanan, G. C., and Drake, T. S. (1978). Comparison of the fractional postcoital test and semen analysis. *Am. J. Obstet. Gynecol.*, **130**, 647–52.

Trimbos-Kemper, G. C., Trimbos, J. B., and van Hall, E. (1984). Pregnancy rates after laparoscopy for infertility. *Eur. J. Obstet. Gynec. Reprod. Biol.*, **18**, 127–32.

Trounson, A. O., Mohr, L. R., Wood, C., and Leeton, J. F. (1982). Effect of delayed insemination on *in vitro* fertilization, culture and transfer of human embryos. *J. Reprod. Fertil.*, **64**, 285–94.

Tsuji, Y., Clausen, H., Nudelman, E., Kaizo, T., Hakomori, S. I., and Isojima, S. (1988). Human sperm carbohydrate antigens defined by an antisperm human monoclonal antibody derived from an infertile woman bearing antisperm antibodies in her serum. *J. Exp. Med.*, **168**, 343–56 (Abstract).

Tulloch, W. S. (1955). Varicocele in subfertility. Results of treatment. *Br. Med. J.*, **2**, 356–8.

Turner, T. T. (1979). On the epididymis and its function. *Invest. Urol.*, 16, 311–21.

Uher, J., Rypacek, F., and Presl, J. (1990). Transport of novel ovum surrogates in the human fallopian tube: a clinical study. *Fertil. Steril.*, 54, 278–82.

Upadhyaya, M., Hibbard, B. M., and Walker, S. M. (1984). Antisperm antibodies and male infertility. *Br. J. Urol.*, 56, 531–6.

Valle, R. F. (1980). Hysteroscopy in the evaluation of female infertility. *Am. J. Obstet. Gynecol.*, 137, 425–31.

Vande Wiele, R. L., Bogumil, J., Dyrenfurth, I., Ferin, M., Jewelewicz, R., Warren, M., *et al.* (1970). Mechanisms regulating the menstrual cycle in women. *Rec. Prog. Hor. Res.*, 26, 63–103.

van Dijk, J. G., Frolich, M., Brand, E. C., and van Hall, E. V. (1979). The 'treatment' of unexplained infertility with danazol. *Fertil. Steril.*, 31, 481–5.

van Noord-Zaadstra, B. M., Looman, C. W., Alsbach, H., Habbema, J. D. F., te Velde, E. R., and Karbaat, J. (1991). Delaying childbearing: effect of age on fecundity and outcome of pregnancy. *Br. Med. J.*, 302, 1361–5.

Verkauf, B. S. (1983). The incidence and outcome of single-factor, multifactorial, and unexplained infertility. *Am. J. Obstet. Gynecol.*, 147, 175–81.

Vermesh, M. and Kletzky, O. A. (1987). Longitudinal evaluation of the luteal phase and its transition into the follicular phase. *J. Clin. Endocrinol. Metab.*, 65, 653–8.

Vermesh, M., Kletzky, O. A., Davajan, V., and Israel, R. (1987). Monitoring techniques to predict and detect ovulation. *Fertil. Steril.*, 47, 259–64.

Vessey, M., Doll, R., Peto, R., Johnson, B., and Wiggins, P. (1976). A long-term follow-up study of women using different methods of contraception—an interim report. *J. Biosoc. Sci.*, 8, 373–427.

Vierikko, P., Kauppila, A., Ronnberg, L., and Vihko, R. (1985). Steroidal regulation of endometriosis tissue: lack of induction of 17-beta hydroxysteroid dehydrogenase activity by progesterone, medroxyprogesterone acetate, or danazol. *Fertil. Steril.*, 43, 218–24.

Vutyavanich, T. and Collins, J. A. (1991). An overview of the Canadian Infertility Therapy Evaluation Study. *J. Soc. Obst. Gyn. Can.*, 13, 29–34.

Wang, C., Chan, S. Y. W., Ng, M., So, W. W. K., Tsoi, W.-L., Lo, T., *et al.* (1988). Diagnostic value of sperm function tests and routine semen analyses in fertile and infertile men. *J. Androl.*, 9, 384–9.

Wathen, N. C., Perry, L., Lilford, R. J., and Chard, T. M. (1984). Interpretation of single progesterone measurement in diagnosis of anovulation and defective luteal phase: observations on analysis of the normal range. *Br. Med. J. (Clin. Res.)*, **288** (6410), 7–9.

Webster, Noah (1983). *Webster's ninth new collegiate dictionary*, p. 307. Thomas Allan and Son, Markham, Ontario.

Weinberg, C. R., Wilcox, A. J., and Baird, D. A. (1989). Reduced fecundability in women with prenatal exposure to cigarette smoking. *Am. J. Epidemiol.*, **129**, 1072–8.

Welner, S., Decherney, A. H., and Polan, M. L. (1988). Human menopausal gonadotropins: a justifiable therapy in ovulatory women with long-standing idiopathic infertility. *Am. J. Obstet. Gynecol.*, **158**, 111–17.

Wentz, A. C. (1980). Endometrial biopsy in the evaluation of infertility. *Fertil. Steril.*, **33**, 121–4.

Wentz, A. C. (1990). Luteal phase inadequacy. In *Infertility, a comprehensive text* (ed. M. M. Siebel), pp. 83–96. Appleton and Lange, Norwalk, Connecticut.

West, C. P., Templeton, A. A., and Lees, M. M. (1982). The diagnostic classification and prognosis of 400 infertile couples. *Infertility*, **5**, 127–44.

Westrom, L. (1975). Effect of acute pelvic inflammatory disease on fertility. *Am. J. Obstet. Gynecol.*, **121**, 707–13.

Westrom, L. (1980). Incidence, prevalence, and trends of acute pelvic inflammatory disease and its consequences in industrialized countries. *Am. J. Obstet. Gynecol.*, **138**, 880–92.

Wiltbank, M. C., Kosasa, S., and Rogers, B. (1985). Treatment of infertile patients by intrauterine insemination of washed spermatozoa. *Andrologia*, **17**, 22–30 (Abstract).

Witkin, S. S., Bongiovanni, A. M., Berkeley, A., Ledger, W. J., and Toth, A. (1984). Detection and characterization of immune complexes in the circulation of infertile women. *Fertil. Steril.*, **42**, 384–8.

Witschi, E. (1948). Migration of the germ cells of human embryos from the yolk sac to the primitive gonadal folds. *Contributions to Embryology*, **32**, 67–80.

Wolff, H. and Schill, W. B. (1985). A modified enzyme-linked immunosorbent assay (ELISA) for the detection of antisperm antibodies. *Andrologia*, **17**, 426–34.

Wood, G., Baker, G., and Trounson, A. (1984). Current status and future prospects. In *Clinical in vitro fertilization* (ed. C. Wood and A. Trounson), pp. 11–26. Springer-Verlag, Berlin.

WHO (World Health Organization) (1983). A prospective multicentre trial of the ovulation method of natural family planning. III. Characteristics of the menstrual cycle and of the fertile phase. *Fertil. Steril.*, 40, 773–8.

WHO (World Health Organization) (1986). Comparative trial of tubal insufflation, hysterosalpingography, and laparoscopy with dye hydro-tubation for assessment of tubal patency. *Fertil. Steril.*, 46, 1101.

WHO (World Health Organization) (1987). *WHO Laboratory manual for the examination of human semen and semen–cervical mucus interaction*, pp. 1–26. Cambridge University Press.

Wright, C. S., Steele, S. J., and Jacobs, H. S. (1979). Value of bromo-criptine in unexplained primary infertility: a double-blind controlled trial. *Br. Med. J.*, 1, 1037–9.

Wright, J., Allard, M., Lecours, A., and Sabourin, S. (1989). Psycho-social distress and infertility: a review of controlled research. *Int. J. Fertil.*, 34, 126–42.

Yanagimachi, R. (1984). Zona-free hamster eggs: their use in assessing fertilizing capacity and examining chromosomes of human spermatozoa. *Gamete Res.*, 10, 187–232.

Yanagimachi, R. (1988). Mammalian fertilization. In *The physiology of reproduction* (ed. E. Knobil, J. D. Neill, L. L. Ewing, C. L. Markert, G. S. Greenwald, and D. W. Pfaff), pp. 135–85. Raven Press, New York.

Yanagimachi, R., Yanagimachi, H., and Rogers, B. J. (1976). The use of zona-free animal ova as a test-system for the assessment of the fertilizing capacity of human spermatozoa. *Biol. Reprod.*, 15, 471–6.

Yanagimachi, R., Lopata, A., Odom, C. B., Bronson, R. A., Mahi, C. A., and Nicolson, G. L. (1979). Retention of biologic characteristics of zona pellucida in highly concentrated salt solution: the use of salt-stored eggs for assessing the fertilizing capacity of spermatozoa. *Fertil. Steril.*, 31, 562–74.

Yen, S. S. C. and Jaffe, R. B. (1986). *Reproductive endocrinology: physiology, pathophysiology, and clinical management*, 2nd edn, pp. 1–806. Saunders, Philadelphia.

Yovich, J. L. and Matson, P. L. (1988). Early pregnancy wastage after gamete manipulation. *Br. J. Obstet. Gynaecol.*, 95, 1120–7.

Yovich, J. L., Stanger, J. D., Kay, D., and Boettcher, B. (1984). *In-vitro* fertilization of oocytes from women with serum antisperm antibodies. *Lancet*, i, 369–70.

Yudin, A. I., Hanson, F. W., and Katz, D. F. (1989). Human cervical mucus and its interaction with sperm: a fine-structural view. *Biol. Reprod.*, 40, 661–71.

Yuzpe, A. A., Gomel, V., and Taylor, P. J. (1986). Endoscopy in the patient with endometriosis. In *Laparoscopy and hysteroscopy in gynecologic practice* (ed. V. Gomel, P. J. Taylor, A. A. Yuzpe, and J. E. Rioux), pp. 111–22. Yearbook Medical Publishers, Chicago.

Zaini, A., Jennings, M. G., and Baker, H. W. (1985). Are conventional sperm morphology and motility assessments of predictive value in sub-fertile men? *Int. J. Androl.*, **8**, 427–35.

Zamboni, L. (1970). Ultrastructure of mammalian oocytes and ova. *Biol. Reprod.*, **2**, 44–63.

Zanchetta, R., Busolo, F., and Mastrogiacomo, I. (1982). The enzyme-linked immunosorbent assay for detection of the antispermatozoal antibodies. *Fertil. Steril.*, **38**, 730–4.

Zavos, P. M. (1985). Seminal parameters of ejaculates collected from oligospermic and normospermic patients via masturbation and at intercourse with the use of a silastic seminal fluid collection device. *Fertil. Steril.*, **44**, 517–20.

Zorn, J. R., Cedard, L., Nessman, C., and Savale, M. (1984). Delayed endometrial maturation in women with normal progesterone levels. *Gynecol. Obstet. Invest.*, **17**, 157–62.

Index